DATE DUE

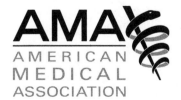

AMERICAN
MEDICAL
ASSOCIATION

D1401903

Executive Vice President, Chief Executive Officer: Michael D. Maves, MD, MBA
Chief Operating Officer: Bernard L. Hengesbaugh
Senior Vice President, Publishing and Business Services: Robert A. Musacchio, PhD
Vice President, Business Products: Anthony J. Frankos
Director, Editorial and Operations: Mary Lou White
Senior Acquisitions Editor: Marsha Mildred
Director, Production and Manufacturing: Jean Roberts
Director, Business Marketing and Communication: Pam Palmersheim
Director, Sales and Strategic Partnerships: J. D. Kinney
Manager, Developmental Editing: Nancy Baker
Project Manager: Katharine Dvorak
Senior Production Specialist: Boon Ai Tan
Senior Print Production Specialist: Ronnie Summers
Marketing Manager: Leigh Bottiger

Library of Congress Cataloging-in-Publication Data

Maximizing billing and collections in the medical practice / by the Coker
    Group ; [editor, Kay Stanley].
        p. ; cm.
    Includes index.
    Summary: "Provide analytical tools and systematic review processes
for the practice administrator to strengthen the practice's business
operations"–Provided by publisher.
    ISBN-13: 978-1-57947-867-4
    ISBN-10: 1-57947-867-0
    1. Medicine—Practice–Finance.   2. Medical offices–Management.
3. Accounts receivable—Management.   4. Medical fees.   I. Stanley,
Kay, 1944– . II. Coker Group.   III. American Medical Association.
    [DNLM: 1. Patient Credit and Collection.   2. Practice Management,
Medical.   3. Fees, Medical.   4. Insurance, Health, Reimbursement.
W 80 M464 2007]
    R728.5.M394 2007
    610.68'3—dc22

                                                             2006032605

BQ13:06-P-043:12/06

CONTENTS

List of Figures, Tables, and Forms   xii
Preface   ix
Acknowledgments   xi
About the Coker Group   xiii

Chapter 1: Getting Ready for a Self-Assessment   1
Gather Data   1
Understand Your Practice Information   3
Perform a Cursory Review   4
Summary   5

Chapter 2: Tracking the Patient Encounter
and Interviewing Front Office Staff   7
Review the Patient Encounter   7
Interview the Front Office Staff   8
Practice manager   9
Receptionist   9
Billing clerk   10
Insurance specialist   11
Summary   11

Chapter 3: Completing the Analysis   13
Accounts Receivable   13
Collection Levels   14
Departmental Administrative Direction
and Leadership   15
Operational Organization   16
Computer Systems and Associated Processes   17
Upgrade the system 18
Establish electronic claims filing   18
Use a lockbox service   18
Department Personnel Training   19
Policies and Procedures Manual   19
Adjustment Process   20
Copayment Collection   21
Patient Education   22
Staffing Levels   22
Management Reports   23
Charge Capture   23
Compliance Plan   26
Internal Controls and Cash Handling   27

Coding   28
Managed Care Information   29
Physical Facility   29
Summary   30

Chapter 4: Setting Up Billing
          and Collections Operations   31
          Identifying Roles and Assigning Responsibilities   31
          Employing the Right People   31
          Establishing Payment Policies and Fees   33
          Using Performance Standards for Collectors   37
          Rewarding Performance Through Bonus Plans   38
          Applying Coding Knowledge   38
          Summary   39

Chapter 5: Getting Paid by the Patient   41
          Collecting at the Time of Service   41
          Offering Discounts for Cash Payments   43
          Confirming and Gathering Copyaments   47
          Recognizing the Importance of Copayments   49
          Collecting from HSAs, HRAs, and Other
             High-Deductible Plans   50
          Establishing Collection Goals   51
          Making the Most of Balance Billing   53
          Understanding Usury Laws and Finance Charges   57
          Charging for No Shows   57
          Summary   58

Chapter 6: Getting Paid by Insurers   61
          Verifying Patient Insurance   62
          Using the Internet   62
          Submitting a Clean Claim   63
             Prebilling   64
             Claims transmission   65
             Payer follow-up   65
             Payment posting   66
             Denial management   66
             Statement generation   66
             Collections   66
             Retrospective and concurrent review   66
          Developing Payer Profiles and Analyses   68
          Dealing with Slow Insurance Payers   73
             Prompt pay laws   74
             Recoupment of payments made by payers   74
          Identifying Incorrect Payments   75
          Automating Requests for Information from
             the Provider   76

Instituting a Follow-up System for Unpaid
or Rejected Claims   77
Appealing Denied Claims   79
Using Software to File an Appeal   79
Understanding the Appeals Process   80
Urgent review   81
Level 1 appeal   81
Level 2 appeal   82
Level 3 appeal   82
Other stages   82
Filing Grievances with the State Insurance
Commission   83
Summary   84

Chapter 7: Getting Paid by Medicare   85
Know What Will and Will Not Be Paid   85
Advance Beneficiary Notice   85
Keep Up with Policy Changes   88
Submit a Clean Claim   89
Use the Medicare Appeals Process   90
First level of appeal: redetermination   90
Second level of appeal: reconsideration   90
Third level of appeal: administrative law judge   91
*Fourth level of appeal: Medicare Appeals
Council review   91*
*Final level of appeal: federal district
court review   92*
Use of Medicare Electronic Data Interchange   92
Pay Attention to Fraud: Compliance Should
Be Part of Everyday Billing Practices   93
Summary   94

Chapter 8: Managing Parallel Payment Systems   95
Manage on the Front End   95
Manage on the Back End   97
Capitation: Verifying Coverage and Monitoring
Utilization   97
Billing for Fee-for-Service Carve-outs   99
Summary   100

Appendix A: Prompt Pay Statutes and Regulations   101

Appendix B: Resources   111

Glossary   113

Index   139

LIST OF FIGURES, TABLES, AND FORMS

Figures

Figure 3-1. Likelihood of Recovery of Accounts Receivable   14
Figure 3-2. Sample Flash Report #1   24
Figure 3-3. Sample Flash Report #2   25
Figure 4-1. Sample Scenario Flowchart   32
Figure 4-2. Sample Front Office Functions   34
Figure 4-3. Sample Business Office Functions   35
Figure 6-1. Claims Processing Flowchart   67

Tables

Table 1-1. Billing and Collections Assessment Checklist   2
Table 3-1. Sample Daily Collections Summary Sheet   27
Table 6-1. Clean Claim Interventions   69
Table 7-1. Sample Chart of Medicare-Covered Services   86
Table 7-2. Medicare Appeals Process   90
Table 8-1. Sample Front Office Managed Care Matrix   96
Table 8-2. Sample Back Office Managed Care Matrix   98

Forms

Form 5-1. Sample Financial Agreement   44
Form 5-2. Collection Success Analysis   52
Form 6-1. Payer Plan Profiles   71
Form 6-2. Payer Organization Profiles   72
Form 6-3. Sample Claim Appeal Letter   81
Form 7-1. Universal Advance Beneficiary Notice   87

Shrinking reimbursements and rising costs for the delivery of health care are compelling practices to be diligent in their billing and collections procedures. Physicians typically are working harder, staying busier, and yet collecting far less than they are entitled to receive for the level of services they are performing. *Maximizing Billing and Collections in the Medical Practice* is written to provide analytical tools and systematic review processes to strengthen the practice's business operations. For the practice administrator, often, a careful review and assessment is just what is needed to find weaknesses in the practice's policies and procedures and to learn where training needs to be conducted among employees. In matters of billing and collections, "the devil is in the details." For example, the hard part of collecting from payers is in the many small details that are required of the claims process. Further, the difficulty in collecting from patients is often in knowing why and how to go about it—that is, what to do and say—and when!

The analytical approach offered as the basis of this book is intended to present concrete, practical information on the many details and requirements of billing and collections. Flowcharts, graphs, and tables illustrate the many steps in the billing and collections process, particularly with third-party payers. It is essential to submit claims for reimbursement correctly—the first time. In addition, it is mandatory to appeal with persistence those claims that are denied.

Further, as the influence of consumer-driven health care intensifies, the medical practice must become increasingly diligent in collecting at the time of service and arranging for payment when accommodations are necessary. Patients will be creative in ways to reduce their payment amounts or delay what they have to pay out of pocket for their health care. The medical practice must be ready to face these challenges, while answering the health care needs of the patient. This book offers some fundamental and key techniques for accomplishing that.

Getting Ready
for a Self-Assessment

The purpose of this book is to present a method of assessment that, when used continually or periodically, will improve practice operations. In a typical medical practice, staff members follow the work routines taught to them by their managers or predecessors. Staff members also have developed methods that make sense to them. Some—in fact, many—of these systems work well. Other systems, however, have become outdated as a result of changes in billing and collections practices forced onto medical practices by the marketplace. The hurried pace of the practice environment often keeps staff members or managers from being able to augment their procedures—even if they know they are flawed.

Because previous routines may no longer be as effective as they were in the past, every practice should conduct periodic assessments of its billing and collections practices to gain insight into the state of affairs. Although it may be preferable to engage an outside reviewer to maintain objectivity, doing so is not necessary. This chapter will help physicians and practice managers gather the information they need to conduct an in-house assessment of its billing and collections practices, understand their practice information, and perform a cursory review of the information.

GATHER DATA

To begin the billing and collections assessment, you will need to review a number of important documents. The first step, therefore, is to gather key practice data and to have it on hand for the steps that follow. Table 1-1 is a billings and collections assessment checklist to use to begin gathering this data.

T A B L E   1-1

Billing and Collections Assessment Checklist

_____ 1. Physician curriculum vitae (CVs) and identification (ID) numbers

_____ 2. A sample superbill or fee ticket

_____ 3. A sample hospital billing information sheet or billing card that is used to document hospital procedures performed during emergency room call and scheduled surgical procedures (ie, a face sheet)

_____ 4. An accounts receivable aging report for the practice (preferably for the past 180+ days)

_____ 5. Accounts receivable by physician

_____ 6. Accounts receivable by payer (reflecting the aging of each plan)

_____ 7. Accounts receivable by patient

_____ 8. Accounts receivable by location (eg, satellite offices)

_____ 9. A collections report documenting gross charges versus net collections and corresponding adjustment rates (by month of current period and previous fiscal year-to-date)

_____ 10. A collections report documenting gross charges versus net collections and corresponding adjustment rates sorted by payer (by month of current period and previous fiscal year-to-date)

_____ 11. Income statement for the most recent period and for the previous fiscal year-to-date

_____ 12. Procedure report by month for the most recent period and for the previous fiscal year-to-date sorted by the top 50 codes

_____ 13. Procedure report (Current Procedural Terminology [CPT®] codes) by month by physician

_____ 14. Procedure report (CPT codes) by month by facility

_____ 15. Tax return for the prior calendar year

_____ 16. A listing of referral sources and corresponding referral numbers, by month, for the most recent period

_____ 17. Sample practice collection letters, if any

_____ 18. A list of hospital participation and corresponding privilege levels

_____ 19. A list of participating payers

_____ 20. A sample of 25 explanations of benefits (EOB) and 5 remittance advice forms (a mixture of clean and unclean claims)

_____ 21. A sample error (rejected claims) report from the electronic claims filing procedure

_____ 22. A sample statement for patient-responsible balances

_____ 23. A description of the practice management and billing software system and its capabilities

_____ 24. A list of staff members and their job descriptions and salaries

_____ 25. Samples of all internal reports currently generated by the practice for a review of billing and collections

_____ 26. Patient demographic data by age and zip code

_____ 27. Copies of all managed care contracts

_____ 28. A copy of the practice fee schedule that lists all codes

_____ 29. A sample patient information sheet

_____ 30. A copy of current Medicare Allowables if the practice participates in Medicare.

The Coker Group expresses appreciation to several reviewers and contributors to this work, namely Susan Childs, FACMPE; Keith Solinsky; and Linda Swadener, FACMPE. Each of these three individuals provided critical thinking and insight from an active administrator's viewpoint of the requirements necessary to improve efficient billing and collections and business operations. Thank you for taking time from your busy schedules to provide input and content.

ABOUT THE COKER GROUP

The Coker Group is a leading national health care consulting firm, with unparalleled expertise in practice management, financial, and technology problem-solving. For over 20 years, Coker has delivered to its clients the best in service, support, and results. Through careful, detailed analysis, Coker's experienced consultants are able to formulate plans and implement realistic, effective strategies. The Coker Group offers services in the following areas:

- Practice management consulting
- Health information technology
- Publishing and education
- Hospital consulting
- Executive recruiting
- Financial services and assistance with financial transactions
- Research and analysis

The Coker Group was founded in 1987 to institute better relations between physicians and hospitals. In those first years, Coker worked closely with hospitals to build the allegiance of physicians on hospital medical staffs, operating mostly through noncontractual relationships.

Over time, still concentrating on physician and hospital relationships, The Coker Group responded to the health care industry's changing needs. They started to operate under formal contracting arrangements on projects involving the research, development, and formation of contracted alliances for hospitals and physicians.

Today, The Coker Group offers a wide variety of health care consulting services across the United States. Thousands of health care organizations have trusted Coker with their success.

Atlanta Office
1000 Mansell Exchange West, Suite 310
Alpharetta, GA 30022
(678) 832-2000

Philadelphia Office
Montgomery Avenue,
1st Floor
Narbeth, PA 19072
(866) 539-3103

(800) 345-5829
www.cokergroup.com

The second step involves conducting interviews with the physicians. Whether the billing and collections assessment was initiated by the physician-owners of a practice; by the employer, such as a health system that owns the practice and employs the physicians; or by employed physicians, it is important to involve the physicians in the process and it is essential to have their cooperation and support.

Note

If the financial statements contain codes, abbreviations, or other information not easily identifiable, it is wise to have a key available that outlines the corresponding meanings of those codes or abbreviations (eg, *MC = Medicare, MD = Medicaid, Physician Code 013 = Dr Smith*). Keep this list nearby during the review process.

Explain the assessment process to the physicians. Set expectations for the assessment and a timeline for completion. Go through the checklist of information with the physicians, and explain each document on the list and how it will be used in the assessment.

Interview the physicians with the expectations of uncovering their specific concerns. Make it possible for them to be introspective and open. For example, a physician may tell you that he or she is busier than ever—seeing more patients, performing more procedures—yet the cash flow may be surprisingly sparse. Or perhaps a physician has noticed unusual or suspect behavior on the part of another staff member that he or she previously has been reluctant to discuss, which may reveal a breakdown in the collection process.

UNDERSTAND YOUR PRACTICE INFORMATION

The documents you gather will provide the information you need to assess the practice. Ensure that all of the documents are together before getting started.

Begin by reviewing the income statement. Often an income statement will point out obvious areas of trouble, such as expenses that are higher than the norm or a revenue shortfall.

Next, review the accounts receivable aging report. Monthly review of this report is an integral part of the billing and collections manager's routine. The report should show the practice's success in collections by payer. Some obvious areas to look at are the percentage of receivables by aging category and the total receivables. Although each specialty may differ to some extent, 85% of your receivables should be current in categories of 30–60 days, 10–12%

current in 61–90 days, and the remainder in 90+ days. Your 90-day balance usually reflects claims for which there was a problem obtaining payment, or reflects a global package that is aging due to an older originating date of service. If possible, try to maintain one date of service so that you can see the true aging of the account.

After reviewing the accounts receivable aging report, look over the report that shows the adjustment rate (ie, gross charges versus net charges). Several sources provide information on acceptable adjustment rates by specialty, such as the American Medical Group Association (AMGA) and the Medical Group Management Association (MGMA). Generally, adjustments to billed charges should not total more than 40%. Again, this can depend upon the practice's specialty and types of services provided. It also depends on your contracts and negotiating power.

Finally, review the collections adjustments. Using benchmarks obtained from sources such as the AMGA, MGMA, and specialty academies, look at the performance standards of other practices. Although these items come at an expense, they are often worthwhile sources as comparables. The specialty academies are beginning to gather this sort of data and will be able to offer it by specialty, as opposed to a volume that addresses appropriate billing and collections levels for all specialties across all regions of the United States.

Next create a chart and mark your position on the chart. Does your practice fall within the 25%, 50%, or 75% range? Typically, you will want to rank in the 50th percentile at a minimum in a heavily managed care market, and at least in the 75th percentile in a low managed care environment.

The objective of this initial exercise is to review the documents from a fresh perspective. Later in this book, we examine each item for the purpose of completing the assessment.

PERFORM A CURSORY REVIEW

Use the billings and assessment checklist in Table 1-1 and the review of your practice information to make a note of each obvious problem. Develop a list of questions. Include the areas that you think may contribute to potential collections problems. Often, your instincts are right. Plan to go back to these questions later, and record your assumptions as answers become available.

Once you have created this list, use it to create an action plan for addressing the problem areas.

SUMMARY

The initial planning of an assessment of the practices' billing and collections process is often the most crucial stage. Gather all relevant materials together and review them. Involve the physician and gather input. Make notes of obvious problems and develop a list of questions to answer. Have sound and pertinent benchmarking statistics at hand so that you can accurately gauge your practice's performance. By conducting objective and periodic assessments, and making appropriate adjustments to your processes, you can maximize and maintain successful results in billing and collections.

chapter 2

Tracking the Patient Encounter and Interviewing Front Office Staff

A patient encounter begins with the first call to the practice by a prospective patient. The collection process also begins at the first call, and the first call is when the success or failure of the collection process is set up. The dialogue that occurs between the patient and the telephone attendant or receptionist during that initial patient contact can determine whether the patient will be cooperative about making sure that the physician is compensated for his or her time. For this reason, it is necessary for those on the front line of patient interaction to develop a stream of consciousness of the importance of their role in the encounter. Ongoing training and assessment will be a means of developing a positive impact in the relationship with the patient and an important aspect in whether the patient understands the responsibility to pay for services.

REVIEW THE PATIENT ENCOUNTER

To assess the billing and collections process as it relates to a patient encounter, it is important to review each step of the patient encounter, starting when a new or established patient calls for an appointment. Write down what the receptionist/scheduler tells the patient and what information is obtained from the patient. Then ask yourself the following questions:

■ Which staff member schedules the appointment?
■ Is complete and accurate demographic information entered into the computer as the call is made?
■ Does the staff member tell a new patient about billing policies and collection procedures?
■ Will the patient arrive at the practice on the day and time of the appointment prepared to pay for the services rendered

using cash, a check, or a credit card, or by submitting an insurance claim?

- Is a brochure describing the practice, the hours of operation, the physician profiles, and billing policies mailed to a new patient? (You may also mail brochures to patients if your billing policies change or if you add a new physician or service.)

- Is a new patient asked to complete a patient information sheet with all relevant guarantor, employer, and demographic information while he or she is at the office? (Using a secure connection, you can offer online registration on your Web site to attain patient information prior to the appointment.)

- How does the front office verify eligibility of coverage for patients with a third-party payer?

- What is the practice's policy on automobile insurance or third-party payers?

- Does the practice scan or make a copy of the patient's insurance card at every patient visit?

- Does the practice accept secondary and tertiary insurance?

If the patient is new to the practice, details about copayments, deductibles, coinsurance, and noncovered services (if not indicated on the patient's insurance plan member identification [ID] card), can be gathered when the patient presents for the encounter and verified while the physician is examining the patient. If the practice is a specialty office, verifying patient payment responsibilities can be obtained while coordinating the referral before the patient visit.

Note

With the proper demographic profile, it is easier to collect the appropriate payment for noncovered items before the patient leaves the office.

INTERVIEW THE FRONT OFFICE STAFF

Interviewing the front office staff can often reveal mistakes in the processes of a patient encounter that can potentially become obstacles to collection. Conducting interviews can also reveal strengths and weaknesses that can later be adjusted to improve the practice's billing and collections procedures. Often, the staff members who are in daily contact with patients have the most information about how to improve current processes. It is advisable to query staff members at least quarterly to find out their ideas for improvement, not just for billing and collections, but for all practice management processes.

Note

Make sure the staff members who answer telephones and receive patients have good communication and listening skills. Instruct them on how to ask the right questions and how to be sensitive to patients—both those who are well and those who are ill. Inspire your employees to view their jobs as problem solvers and gatherers of information rather than as appointment bookers or gatekeepers.

Practice manager

Quite possibly, the practice administrator or manager is conducting the review of the practice's billing and collections procedures. Nevertheless, all functions must be examined for efficiencies, even if this entails self-examination.

Begin by chronicling (or having the practice manager chronicle) a patient encounter from start to finish—from the time the patient contacts the practice by telephone to set up an appointment, all the way through the completion of the medical record and the resolution of any outstanding accounts receivable. The practice manager should record in writing all of the steps that occur. Putting procedures on paper is one way of identifying where loopholes exist and where improvements can be made to benefit business operations.

Receptionist

The receptionist or the staff member who answers the telephone to make patient appointments is often the first person who discusses anything to do with the practice, the patient, and the financial relationship between the two. Ensure that the receptionist is well aware of all of the financial parameters established by the practice and is comfortable and confident talking about them.

Let us start with the person who answers the telephone and schedules the appointments. Typically, this staff member's role is to listen to the patient's request for a time slot that is convenient and to match that time with available slots in the appointment schedule. Although this is the most important first step in any patient encounter, it is only the first step in setting up an accurate patient process.

Once the appointment is scheduled, it is important to collect information that will make it easier for the patient to participate in the practice's billing and collection process. Often, if this part of the process is not completed, the rest of the process suffers.

We recommend using the initial telephone call to gather information about the patient's insurance or managed care plan, copayments, deductibles, coinsurance, and guarantor information. These particulars then can be verified with the plan provider by phone or by Internet before the patient arrives for the appointment. When accurate enrollment data is housed in the practice, the patient can be matched to the enrollment data, and coverage can be verified.

In addition, coverage has already been verified when the patient arrives at the practice, speeding up the process of checking in the patient. If there is an information sheet upon arrival at the medical practice, each new patient should complete it. This should provide information about the patient's address, employer, guarantor, emergency contact information, primary and secondary insurance, subscriber, and so on. Each established patient should be asked when registering with the office if his or her address has changed on any of the insurance information.

Some practices post patient registration forms on the practice's Web site for patients who are willing or prefer to provide information online. This speeds up the registration process prior to the patient's arrival and reduces the time needed to fill out or update demographic information or medical history. Expect this trend to grow in the future as more and more patients use the Internet and technology for communication purposes.

Note
Tell new patients about your payment policy at the time you set the appointment. Mail a printed policy to confirm the time of appointment, or hand the policy to the patient upon the patient's arrival.

Billing clerk

The billing clerk is usually responsible for handling the patient's financial information once the encounter has culminated; the copayment, deductible, or coinsurance has been collected; and the patient has left the premises. Usually, the billing clerk sees the patient encounter information and verifies the information on it. For example, the billing clerk (preferably, a person experienced and certified in medical coding) checks to make sure the patient encounter is accurately coded so that the encounter will result in a clean claim. Traditionally, a *clean* claim is a claim that is processed without incident and paid appropriately based on a managed care contracted rate of reimbursement or other standard payment arrangement. An *unclean* claim results in an explanation of benefits that denies the billing of an encounter and documents this rejec-tion with applicable reason codes. (In larger practices, denied claims are usually handled by a qualified coder or by the payment poster.) In addition, the billing clerk will also ensure that the claim is sent to the payer in a timely fashion after the encounter (ie, between 24 and 48 hours after the date of service).

Note
Only the required patient information should be submitted and not the patient's complete medical records.

Insurance specialist

Traditionally, an insurance specialist participates in the billing and collections process once a claim has been sent to the payer for payment and either a payment has been received or there is correspondence about the claim. Depending on the size of the practice, insurance specialists are usually organized by payer or physician, and they follow up on claims submitted to the payers for which they are responsible. For example, an insurance special-ist assigned to Medicare follows up on all outstanding claims for Medicare patients and handles correspondence requiring further medical record information or information about the encounter.

SUMMARY

A close look at the patient encounter will often reveal strengths and weaknesses and opportunities for improvement in the billing and collections procedures. In addition, the front office staff has a responsibility toward the patient and the patient's participation in the practice's billing and collections process. It is often helpful to periodically interview each staff member to ascertain whether changes to the billing and collections process should be made on the basis of patient demographic changes, managed care partici-pation changes, provider changes within the practice, or any other augmentations to the practice management function.

Interviewing staff members is often the best way to reveal prob-lems in the billing and collections process. If you can constantly improve the efficiency of this flow of information, you can often preclude an increase in outstanding accounts receivable. Through careful interviews with the practice staff at the various points of encounter, the astute manager can offer suggestions for improve-ment in communications and guidance of the staff for each step with the patient.

chapter 3

Completing the Analysis

U se the data you collected in Table 1-1 in Chapter 1 to obtain an overview of the practice's billing and collections process. In this chapter we take a look at and provide recommendations for improvement in each of the following categories: accounts receivable, collection levels, departmental administrative direction and leadership, operational organization, computer systems and associated processes, department personnel training, policies and procedures manual, adjustment process, copayment collection, patient education, staffing levels, management reports, charge capture, compliance plan, internal controls and cash handling, coding, managed care information, and physical facility. The conclusions you draw from this analysis will form the plan for improving the practice's billing and collections process.

ACCOUNTS RECEIVABLE

In Chapter 1 we describe the benefits of using benchmarks to compare or assess your billing and collections process. Using benchmarks obtained from the American Medical Group Association (AMGA), the Medical Group Management Association (MGMA), or the appropriate specialty society, plot your practice's accounts receivables against national norms for your specialty. Then ask the following questions:

- Are the levels of the practice greater than normal? If so, what is the variance?
- Where are the balances in the aging categories? Account balances that are at or above 180 days are difficult to collect. (See Figure 3-1 for an illustration of the diminishing likelihood of collections as the account ages.)
- What classifications of balances are in the past-due categories? How many balances are categorized as self-pay? Accounts classified as "self-pay," which are patients who are either uninsured or covered by insurance plans the practice does not participate in, are usually the most difficult to collect. Also, some balances are the patient's responsibility after insurance claims have been paid.

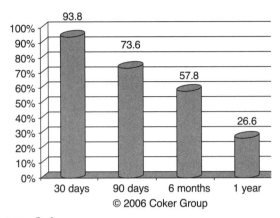

FIGURE 3-1

Likelihood of Recovery of Accounts Receivable

Some remedies can help with the typical problems an accounts receivable analysis reveals. To begin, appoint an internal staff member, a billing service, or outsource the daily operations. The practice manager should have specific, realistic, and attainable accounts receivable target goals and should have the authority to make staffing changes to improve efficiency and increase collections in order to reduce accounts receivable levels.

Next, devise a management reporting system that provides basic information about cash collections and accounts receivable levels. The reports should be run frequently and actual results and predetermined targets should be compared. The reports should be given to the physicians on a monthly basis to review. Also, update the billing and collections computer software to improve efficiency of claims processing and collection activities.

Next, create a task force of experienced collection personnel to reduce accounts receivable levels. Beginning with the 90-day category, work on all accounts of any amount. Then work on only the larger accounts in the older aging categories (ie, more than 90 days past due). Give task force members an incentive to achieve above-average collection results. (Avoid turning these balances over to a collection agency at this point.)

The longer an account goes uncollected the less likely it is to be collected. Figure 3-1 illustrates this principle.

COLLECTION LEVELS

What is the practice's gross collection percentage? How does this number compare with a normal gross collection percentage for other practices in its specialty? As indicated earlier in this chapter, benchmarks for these comparisons can be obtained through the AMGA, MGMA, and specialty society organizations.

Interview the insurance specialist in the practice to answer the following questions:

- What is the policy for account follow-up?
- How often are patient statements sent?
- Does the statement reflect adjustments for payments made by insurance payers?
- Does the statement identify who makes the payments or whether an insurance or patient amount is still due?
- Are statements sent out when only insurance amounts are due?
- Can statement messages be printed upon demand, predetermined, customized, or selectively withheld?

If collection levels are too low based on gross collection percentages, begin by streamlining the insurance specialist's routines to reduce the volume of nonaccount follow-up activities. Establish a collections group that has the primary responsibility of collecting all patient-responsible balances that are aged more than 60 days. The collections group could form the basis of a regular function within the billing and collections department.

Note

Collection of all insurance accounts should remain with the insurance specialist regardless of account aging.

Modify the standard patient statement so that it is used only when the entire balance due is the patient's responsibility. For cases when insurance copayments, deductibles, coinsurance, or noncovered balances are involved, generate a specific patient statement, withholding the standard messages and adding customized collection messages to correspond with the account status. Also, print outstanding balances on the encounter form to alert the provider and other staff members to route the patient for financial counseling before leaving the practice.

DEPARTMENTAL ADMINISTRATIVE DIRECTION AND LEADERSHIP

Effective management and leadership are key to a successful billing and collections department. The central business office manager must function as a leader and a motivator. He or she should be aware of the status of the accounts receivable, days in accounts receivable, and collection percentage for the area of responsibility. He or she should also monitor all activity that goes on in the department, use motivational techniques and incentives, and keep an eye on workloads and accomplishments of the staff. The central business office manager should be regarded as a knowledgeable resource in billing and collections methods. He or she should also be known for giving credit to others and acknowledging their value.

The central business office manager, who is responsible for all daily operations, should have specific attainable accounts receivable goals. This manager should have the authority to make staffing changes that will improve departmental efficiency in increasing collections and reducing accounts receivables.

By recognizing staff members for a job well done when goals are achieved, the central business office manager can inspire staff members by providing recognition for maintaining heavy workloads, accomplishing above average collections, or reducing accounts receivable levels. Each staff member should have a measurable, reasonable, and attainable goal and should receive recognition and reward for attaining or exceeding that goal. The incentives can be monetary or promotional, such as gift certificates, coffee mugs, or practice-specific certificates of achievement.

The central business office manager should also institute an incentive plan for all members of the department to encourage them to exceed goals. For example, if the front office staff has an incentive as well, they will be motivated to get correct patient insurance information up front and to check eligibility. The central business office manager should also receive an incentive that is a significant component of his or her compensation plan.

OPERATIONAL ORGANIZATION

Problems and inefficiencies often result from assigning too many functions to a single staff member. For example, if an insurance specialist is responsible for a specified physician's billing and collection from claims generation through both insurance and patient-responsible balance follow-up, it is unlikely that sufficient time will be available for daily routine billing functions in addition to collection functions.

Typically, insurance specialists do not have time to work on the accounts receivable list for collections. When time is available, they must focus on the 180-day category or the oldest balances first. The 180-day category is the least likely to be collected, however. As a result, the greatest amount of time is spent on efforts that will be the least productive.

To improve operational organization, instruct insurance specialists to work on insurance accounts in all aged categories. Remove or reassign mundane processing tasks, such as reviewing the daily patient visit list. Institute electronic claims filing to reduce the volume of claims that must be manually scanned to verify completeness. Electronic claims filing also eliminates the need for the insurance specialist to fold the claim, stuff the envelope, and mail the claim to the insurance company—manual tasks that are routine, clerical in nature, and do not require specialized knowledge.

COMPUTER SYSTEMS AND ASSOCIATED PROCESSES

A look at the practice's billing and collection process will show whether the process is labor-intensive or automated. Review the materials listed in Table 1-1 in Chapter 1 that you collected and note the following:

- Is the billing and collection process well organized?
- Does the process require manual intervention to ensure continued processing information?
- How much time is being spent on manual applications, such as copying checks?
- To what degree are claims being filed electronically?
- How well does the information system function? Is it reliable, or is it prone to lock up?
- How functional are the information system's screen fields for capturing information?
- Are electronic claims being filed for all payers? What is the percentage of claims being dropped to paper, and why?
- Is scanning technology being used for encounter form input?
- Is electronic remittance posting being used for Medicare and other payers?
- Does the practice use a lockbox service through a financial institution?
- Are explanation of benefits (EOB) scanned into a document imaging system for easy retrieval?
- What plans are in the works for upgrading the electronic billing and collections system?

- Are all relevant reports/tools provided by the practice management system being used?
- Is there an effective training system in place for employees? How do you measure the effectiveness of the training?

The registration staff collects and accurately enters the required patient demographic and health plan coverage information into the practice management database. The registration staff must be thoroughly trained to enter the required health plan data; an incorrect keystroke or placement of information in the wrong field may result in a health plan claim denial. If the registration staff overlooks or enters just one number or letter in the policyholder's identification number incorrectly, the health plan will not be able to identify the policyholder and the result will be a claim denial. It is essential for the practice management system to be functional and for the hardware to support the functions of the software. Otherwise, you will need to upgrade your system.

Upgrade the system

Upgrade the computer system and technological processes to improve billing and collections functions. An upgraded computer system should include a powerful, effective, and reliable practice management and billing and collections program that is or will be compatible with your existing software. By improving your system, your staff will have more time to complete their other responsibilities.

Establish electronic claims filing

Establishing electronic claims and remittance filing for as many payers as possible, including Medicare, will save staff members a considerable amount of time. Consider using a commercial clearinghouse service for claims that are not submitted directly to the payer through your practice management system or through your payer's Web site. Many of these vendors also include a "claim-scrubbing" service to aid in clean claims processing.

Note

Be sure to verify that the "claim-scrubber" software does not change reported codes without your knowledge or apply payer claims edits that may not be appropriate.

Use a lockbox service

Contract with a financial institution for a lockbox service if the volume of payments warrants it. A "lockbox" service refers to a service that can help your practice streamline Health Insurance

Portability and Accountability Act of 1996 (HIPAA)-compliant mail processing and same-day check deposits.

Here's how a lockbox service works: A practice routes its mail to the lockbox service. The bank or other financial institution will receive payments, copy the checks, deposit them to the proper account, and send deposit information daily via a secure, encrypted Web site.

Note

Before deciding to use a lockbox service, ensure that the volume of payments is such that it would be a cost-sharing measure to implement such a service. Most lockbox services are costly. Make an all-out effort to catch up on posting EOBs, even if doing so requires hiring temporary employees for data input.

DEPARTMENT PERSONNEL TRAINING

When computer hardware and software are replaced, it is necessary to train staff members to use the new program or technology. Training includes teaching staff members how to capture demographic and insurance data for consistency in submitting clean insurance claims. It also includes the most efficient way to post and balance charges and payments, file maintenance functions, and cross-training.

Note

Conduct the training away from the office if possible so that staff members can concentrate on learning the new software. Otherwise, the staff members may be continually pulled out of or interrupted during the training.

Training should begin with an initial training cycle for all personnel. Two months later, hold a follow-up training session. Include all staff members, including those working in satellite offices and business sites for the practice. Provide additional training to staff members who have high input error rates, with special attention to checking or proofing for errors. Adjust staffing assignments and workflow to accomplish accurate and timely data input. Establish and reinforce performance parameters and goals with positive financial incentives.

POLICIES AND PROCEDURES MANUAL

A policies and procedures manual is essential to the smooth operation of any medical practice, particularly in its billing and collections department. Without written policies, the department is certain to be plagued with inconsistencies and questionable processes.

The questions to ask about a policies and procedures manual include the following:

- Is a written manual of policies and procedures in place?
- Who is responsible for keeping the manual up to date?
- How often are the policies updated?
- Who is responsible for enforcing the policies once they are in place?

Develop (or update, if a manual is already in place) a billing and collections policies and procedures manual in concert with the implementation of new management software. The manual should include instructions on every function. It should cover special situations, such as reinstatement of adjustments when payments are received from secondary payers; reversal of write-offs; refund processes; application of credit balances to prior or subsequent patient visits; and so on. The manual should also specify the periodic management reports that are required, including those used to monitor departmental performance. In addition, develop a financial policy to mail to patients before the first visit or to hand to them when they come into the office for the encounter.

Finally, enforcement of policies and procedures necessarily follows establishment. What good is it to have a credit policy, for example, that is ignored or disregarded?

ADJUSTMENT PROCESS

Adjusting charges for contractually discounted payments is an important step in the billing and collections function. The adjustment process is significant for the practice's success and viability. To be effective, routines must be simple.

Contractual adjustment routines, corrections to patient accounts, and charge or posting error reversals should not be confused with other types of adjustments, such as refund requests, bad debt write-offs, collection referrals, and professional courtesies. It is important to differentiate the types of balances that require approval. Refunds, contractual adjustments, and bad debt and collection adjustment processes should be separate and distinct.

To be able to judge the appropriateness of payments and adjustments, staff members must be aware of the contracted amounts for various payers under managed care agreements. This will ensure that insurance-generated EOB are accurate in relation to the contracted fees. Staff members who post payments to accounts should use a matrix that lists the contracted fees for the most common

Current Procedural Terminology (CPT®) codes so that reimbursements can be compared with the contracted amounts. Many practice management programs can also automatically post the adjustment when the payer's allowed amounts are built into the system.

Adjustment codes and write-offs that correlate to the specific adjustments should be set up in the billing system in order to track how adjustments are being made. In addition, approvals for contractual adjustments should be made by the billing and collections manager responsible for the collection ratio and accounts receivable levels. The practice manager and the physicians should monitor the adjustment procedures monthly.

COPAYMENT COLLECTION

Copayments represent significant revenue to the medical practice and should be regarded as a mandatory part of the patient encounter. A typical practice generates $15,000 to $30,000 in revenue from copayments per physician per year. Failure to collect the copayments, deductibles, and coinsurance from the patient when they are due may be a violation of the typical payer contract.

Most patients are expected to make payments—either copayments or patient-responsible portions of estimated charges—during the encounter. Each patient should be asked to pay past-due balances or to arrange a payment plan for paying off the balances.

A billing and collections assessment should include the following questions about the practice's collection of copayments and other patient-responsible balances:

- If the patient's insurance coverage includes a copayment, is the patient asked to make the payment when presenting for the encounter?
- For patients in indemnity plans, is collecting patient-responsible portions routine at checkout?
- Does the front desk attempt to collect past due balances?
- How are health savings accounts (HSAs) and other high-deductible plans approached?

Recommendations for improvement in cash flow and reduction of accounts receivable require asking for money at the time of service. *Collect copayments at check-in.* Patients expect to make this payment, which can be paid by cash, check, an HSA debit card, or credit card. Also institute a procedure for collecting past-due balances at check-in. Notifications of past-due balances may involve flagging the charge ticket with a special sticker, creating a place on the charge ticket area, or placing notes in the note or alert area in the practice management system.

All staff members should be trained in basic collection procedures. Practices cannot afford to let patients leave the office without paying for services or arranging for payment. Special circumstances should be handled privately by an experienced collections specialist.

Although many patients may prefer to pay patient-responsible balances after the physician receives the insurance payment, it is reasonable to ask for payment when patient deductibles have not been met.

PATIENT EDUCATION

Patient education is key to collecting for services. In addition to making sure that your patients know your billing and collection policies through notifications, your Web site, and in your practice brochures, you can also educate patients through signage. Consider posting a sign at the front desk stating that copayments are due at the time of service.

Physicians should always refer patients with payment problems or questions to the practice manager to handle. The physician should never say, "Don't worry about it" to the patient who expresses concerns about paying for services. The patient interprets this as permission from the physician not to pay. In referring the patient to the practice manager, the physician–patient clinical relationship is protected. No financial factors are in the way.

STAFFING LEVELS

Achieving an appropriate billing and collections staffing level is difficult at best. Assessment includes reviewing the practice's workload, processes, and level of automation. In assessing the practice's staffing level, consider the following questions:

- How many full-time employees or full-time equivalents are assigned to the billing and collections department?
- What are the benchmarks for staffing according to the AMGA, MGMA, and specialty society data?
- Are staff members keeping up with their workload, or are they asked to work overtime on a regular basis? Are they currently behind on their tasks?
- What expectations are set for billing and collections ratios, if any?

- Are there established deadlines for specific follow-up, such as month end?
- What incentives, if any, are in place to promote objectives?

If the department is not keeping up with its tasks and is behind in the billing and collections process, engage a temporary employee to assist or ask a staff member from a different area to help out. This may entail after-hours work on weekends or during evenings. Review procedures to eliminate unnecessary steps and inefficiencies. Offer incentives for meeting billing and collection goals to reduce past-due accounts receivable and improve collection rates.

MANAGEMENT REPORTS

Management reports are vital to the practice's revenue stream and cash flow. Crucial management reports such as aged insurance claims pending, open claims, and insurance-specific aged receivables help management assess the practice's financial position and manage billings and collections. Access to and use of data is another area for assessment. Following are questions to consider:

- How often are reports generated and how are they used?
- What other reports are available through the information system? How would they help track progress as well as improve the billing and collections process?

Sample "Flash Reports" that provide a quick view of the practice's performance for the month are shown in Figures 3-2 and 3-3.

It is important to determine the practice's reporting requirements. Some examples of helpful reports are CPT code activity count, amount billed and collected, accounts receivable, and collection ratios.

It is also important to ensure that the proper level of software technology is available for the practice. And ensure that the billing and collections department manager is capable of training staff members on report writing features and report analysis.

CHARGE CAPTURE

Reviewing the charge capture procedures is another fundamental area of billing and collections assessment. A great deal of revenue can be lost if patient encounters take place and procedures are performed that are not listed on encounter forms, and if the information from the forms (such as laboratory testing) does not make it to the billing system. An assessment should include the following questions:

Flash Report

	Goal	Current Month	Previous Month	Year-To-Date
Gross Charges (Billings)				
Adjustments				
Net Charges				
Net Collections				
Total Over head Ratio (Total nonphysician expenses + average monthly net charges or collections)				
New Patients				
Total New Patients				
Collections Percentage (Fee-for-service cash collections/fee-for-service charges)				
Profit <Loss> (Cash Basis) (Collections minus expenses)				
Net Income Percentage (Total net income + collections)				

©2006 The Coker Group

FIGURE 3-2
Sample Flash Report #1

Flash Report

Month: _____

Total Charges	
Adjustments	
Net Charges	
Total Receipts	
Bad Debts (W/Os)	
Total Patients Seen	
Total New Patients Seen	
Daily Average	
Collection Ratio	
Accounts Receivable	
Average Per Patient Charge	
Average Per Patient Cost	
Total Monthly Expenses—Nonprovider	
Total Monthly Expenses—Provider	
Net Income—Preprovider Expense	
Net Income—Postprovider Expense	

©2006 The Coker Group

F I G U R E 3-3

Sample Flash Report #2

- What is the control system for encounter forms? Are they prenumbered, automatically numbered, or not numbered?
- What are the processes for capturing hospital charges? (This is a significant potential area for lost revenue.)
- Is a cross-check system in place?

Institute an automatic encounter form control system, such as prenumbering or automated numbering. Implement an audit control to ensure that all encounter forms are submitted daily. This can be done by comparing the daily patient schedule with the numbered encounter forms. See if the hospital can print a list of your practice's patients counted in the daily census. Implement a charge capture audit process at the CPT code service level. Implement a cross-check of hospital and surgery charge capture by comparing outside source documents with internal billing documents. Conduct periodic random audits to ensure that all charges are captured and billed.

COMPLIANCE PLAN

Having a compliance plan is strongly encouraged to avoid being charged with Medicare fraud and abuse. Although not yet required by law, having an established compliance plan in place is a good defensive strategy. An assessment of the practice's current compliance plan should include the following questions:

- Is a compliance plan in place to ensure against Medicare fraud and abuse? If so, what does the plan entail?
- What level of training do physicians and staff members receive about compliance issues and the vulnerability of the practice?
- Is training documented in your employees' personnel files?
- Does your compliance plan include an annual coding audit conducted by an outside entity?

If preliminary or existing documents are in place, review and update them for presentation to senior management and physicians. Once final or revised documents are approved, implement and integrate the plan into the daily operations of the practice and into the policies and procedures of the billing and collections department. Conduct an annual training refresher program, and annually review compliance with antifraud statutes. Consider engaging an outside consultant to assist in the completion and review of the compliance plan.

Note

Every practice should develop and circulate a plan and train staff members about compliance. Every member of the staff should know the penalties for Medicare fraud and abuse.

INTERNAL CONTROLS AND CASH HANDLING

Setting up internal controls for handling payments and cash is mandatory for a medical practice. There are many opportunities for payments to disappear unless controls are in place that limit the likelihood of theft. Part of a billing and collections assessment must focus on the way payments are handled. Some of the important questions to ask about operation and management of incoming cash and payments concern how and when deposits are made, posted, and recorded. Deposit checks and cash payments daily, unless the amounts are so small they do not warrant the effort. Prepare a deposit slip every day, and show a total for that day. If you skip a day, make two deposits the next day. This verifies that all funds received on a given day were deposited. Record each receivable separately on the deposit slip. This provides a good audit trail and serves as proper documentation for posting the receivable. Posting reports back up the deposit slip. Copy each insurance check, and attach the copy to the EOB. Copy each patient check and cash and attach it to a Daily Collections Summary Worksheet. (See Table 3-1 for a sample worksheet.) Enter the check number for bulk checks. This allows a particular check (or cash payment) to match the EOB that comes with it. It also provides a way to track payments, if needed. Also, copying the actual bills used to pay establishes that the money was collected if it later turns up "missing."

Other income paid to physicians, such as honoraria, rental income, interest income, and other fees for nonmedical services, should not be included in the practice deposits. Maintain a log to track these payments as they are received. Give the physicians a copy and retain another in the accounting department for record-keeping purposes. Any income not related to patients' fees (eg, fees for making copies of medical records) should be deposited into the practice's operating account and must be posted to the daily journal to reconcile charges and receipts and to prevent overstatement of the collection rate at month and year end.

TABLE 3-1

Sample Daily Collections Summary Sheet

Date	Patient Account #	Last Name	Check #	Payer	Total Amount Received
10/12/00	123456	Smith	2345	Self	$0255.00
10/12/00	123457	Jones	222	Cigna	$1200.34
10/12/00	123458	Brown	1427	Cigna	$0556.02

Manage cash flow on a daily basis. Use a basic summary sheet to track cash flow as follows:

Beginning balance + Current day deposits − Current day disbursements = Ending balance

Reconcile the bank statement and financial statement book balance each month to be certain of an accurate cash flow. Look at trends to anticipate cash inflow and outflow. Disbursements and reimbursements should be predictable. Unexpected changes should be a signal that investigation is needed.

A system of internal checks and balances helps preclude innocent errors and deliberate fraud. The key is to separate the handling of cash from the accounting records. One staff member receives the cash and checks; another posts it to the books; and a third deposits it in the checking account. It is recommended that checking account reconciliation be performed by a designated staff person or outsourced to an outside accounting firm.

When the volume of checks warrants it, another alternative to handling the accounting practices in-house is to use the bank's lockbox service. Payments are mailed directly to the lockbox address and deposited as received. The bank then sends deposit amounts and copies of checks to the practice for posting to patients' accounts. This increases security and provides an additional cross-check for payment posting. For example, a report should be run daily of total charges and total payments. A different person should run a calculator tape off of the charge tickets of charges and payments. Each report should then be given to the practice manager to review.

CODING

Procedural and diagnostic coding for procedures, services, and diagnosis must be accurate. A billing and collections assessment should include an audit to ensure compliance and appropriate revenue. The questions to ask are as follows:

- Who codes procedures?
- Who reviews the coding of procedures?
- By what means is coding information transmitted to the billing mechanism?
- Is insurance coverage verified in advance of procedures and services? Do problems occur as a result of precertification or lack of coverage?

- Is there a way to list diagnosis to match procedures and labs to ensure appropriate reimbursement?

Conduct periodic audits of the complete coding process through a procedural coding analysis to ensure compliance and appropriateness of fees. Maintain detailed information on the peculiarities of each payer, and meet their specific requirements and variances according to the contractual agreement.

MANAGED CARE INFORMATION

Practices frequently lose money because of a lack of information about the specifics of managed care contracts and the requirements of each plan. The billing and collections department must have current information for providers about each plan, the contracted fees for the most common CPT codes, medical payment policies, and coverage and billing procedures. An assessment of the practice's managed care information should focus on the following questions:

- What information is at hand about each plan? How is it updated?
- Does the information include the name of a plan service representative for each plan?
- How are appeals handled?
- Is a fee schedule attached to each contract?
- How is this information communicated to the staff?

Note

Contracted rates should be input into the practice management/billing system (if available) to assist in tracking inaccurate payment amounts.

Develop a binder for each health plan that includes the contracted fees for the most common CPT codes, coverage, and billing procedures. Maintain a list of problems with this plan to be discussed during renegotiation of the contract. Provide the receptionist and clinical staff at each practice location with a requirement matrix. Maintain updates about provider applications in process, and monitor them at least weekly, reporting results to the billing office and to the physician(s).

PHYSICAL FACILITY

Working space for the billing and collections function is often limited by the physical facility. Noise levels are usually high as there are typically several conversations taking place within a small area. An assessment of the billing and collections department should include observations on space limitations and recommendations for improvements. If privacy, noise, or overcrowding are issues that cannot be resolved, consider relocating the billing and collections department to another location. Distribute telephone headsets to staff members for conducting calls that require concentration. Use space efficiently for office equipment such as scanners, copiers, files, and so on.

SUMMARY

Most assessments of the billing and collections functions of a medical practice will reveal both strengths and weaknesses in operations. Successful operations have effective leadership, systems, policies, processes, technology, and reporting. The observations and recommendations listed in this chapter are a foundation for improving the billing and collections department.

chapter 4

Setting Up Billing and Collections Operations

As part of the assessment process for billing and collections, the practice manager or other staff member who is doing the assessment should go through the exercise of setting up the billing and collections process as if it did not previously exist. Often, pretending that the process is not currently in place and taking the opportunity to start anew will allow fresh thinking. You may end up creating a billing and collections process that is very distinct from the one in place, or you may just change parts of the process.

IDENTIFYING ROLES AND ASSIGNING RESPONSIBILITIES

The first step in setting up the billing and collections process is to identify the personnel who participate in it. These staff members most likely have other roles in practice management, but some parts of their job descriptions pertain to billing and collections. New employees are also a good resource as they are looking at your system with "new eyes." They can often spot "holes" within protocols as well as have ideas on additional procedures that may indeed need improvement. A useful way to begin is to create a flowchart that shows how a patient moves through the practice and how information about that patient is retrieved. Figure 4-1 illustrates a flowchart that describes a practice's current organization and processes.

EMPLOYING THE RIGHT PEOPLE

The key to successful billing and collections is employing the right people. Finding personnel who have the correct skills is often the most difficult part of setting up an efficient process. Start your assessment of the personnel who support the billing and collections process by making a list of all of the staff members who participate in it. Remember to list staff members whose main responsibilities are not billing and collections but who have responsibilities related to the function, such as the practice's telephone receptionist.

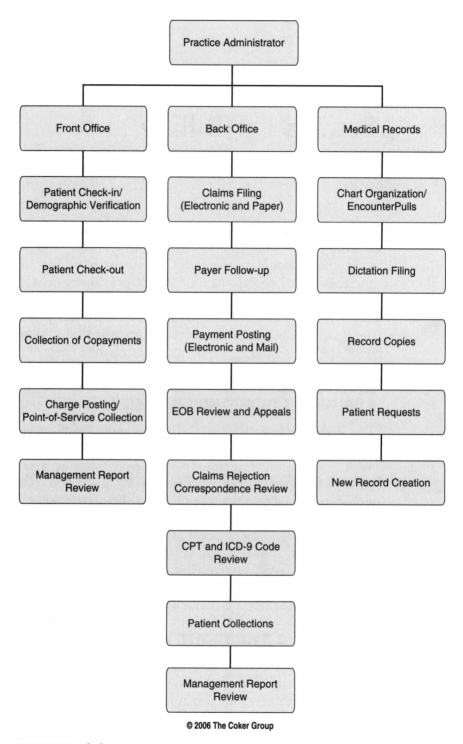

© 2006 The Coker Group

FIGURE 4–1

Sample Scenario Flowchart

When you have made the list, add the functions staff members perform that support billing and collections data gathering and process improvement. Objectively assess whether the staff members you have identified indeed have the right skills for the tasks. For example, a traditional receptionist is crucial to the point-of-service (POS) collections process. Therefore, he or she must possess the following skill set:

- a pleasant, yet direct communication style;
- the ability to communicate with patients regarding their health care coverage;
- the ability to communicate regarding the collection of copayments and past-due balances;
- an understanding of the necessity of gathering all relevant demographic information; and
- strong attention to detail, such as accurate recording of social security or referral numbers.

Ask yourself whether each staff member understands the value of his or her participation in the process. Most employees do not understand that they participate in a process and how important their one function is to the larger process. For example, a medical records clerk may assume that his or her task is simply one of filing. He or she may not understand how essential the documentation surrounding a patient's encounter is to the overall practice.

Following your assessment, you may want to reorganize your front office and business office functions. Figures 4-2 and 4-3 outline front and business office functions, which may be used as a suggestion for front and business office organization, respectively.

ESTABLISHING PAYMENT POLICIES AND FEES

A necessary part of assessing a billing and collections process is to determine whether there are policies and controls in place that efficiently garner payment information and actual payments from patients. The assessment also evaluates whether those payments are proportionate with the time and effort of providers and staff members who support the patient encounter.

If your practice does not have a billing and collections policies and procedures manual, it is recommended you create one. A manual will help you change the billing and collections processes. It also serves as excellent ongoing training and support for staff members when they have questions.

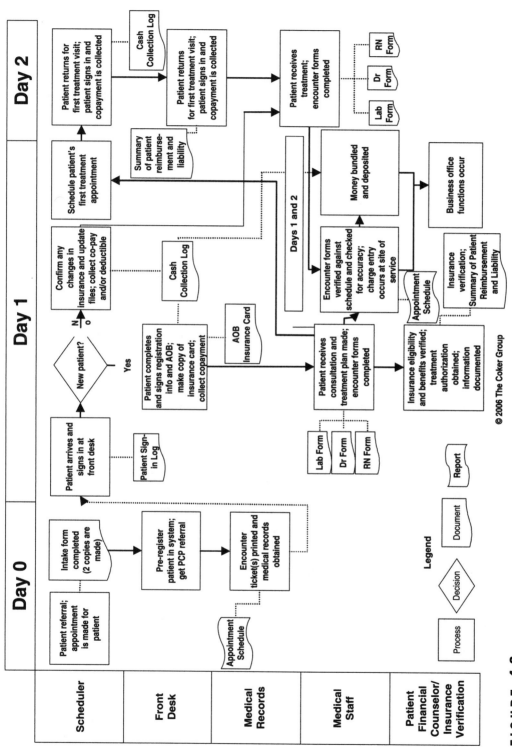

FIGURE 4-2

Sample Front Office Functions

AOB indicates assignment of benefits; PCP, primary care physician

© 2006 The Coker Group

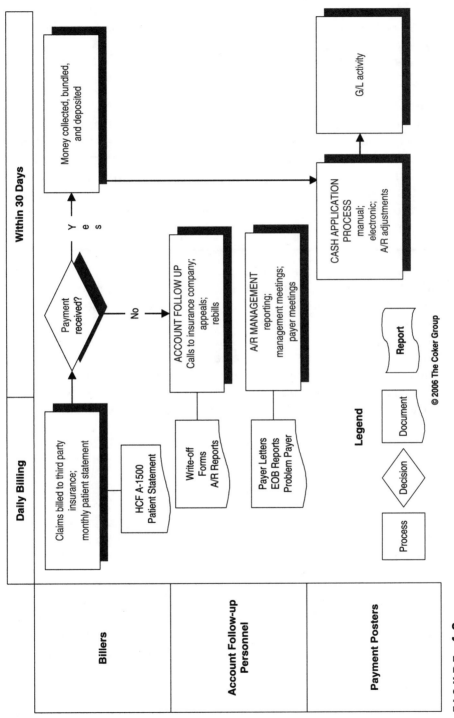

FIGURE 4-3

Sample Business Office Functions

Note: A highlighted shape refers to a process that is not always necessary.

A/R indicates accounts receivable; EOB, explanation of benefits; G/L, general ledger.

35

NOTE

As consultants, we frequently encounter employees who tell us that policies are not in writing. They say that the practice manager has verbally communicated the policies and procedures. On further examination, we discover that each staff member who articulates the policies and procedures relates them quite differently. A written format helps ensure adherence to policies and averts inconsistencies in communication of the policies.

Identifying the correct charges or fees for professional services is often difficult. It does not have to be. Several associations publish fee data that can be compared with the fees charged in your practice. In addition, data is available that supports recommended benchmarks for specialty fees by geographic regions of the United States. These data can help you compare your practice's fees with what other specialists or nonspecialists in your geographic region are charging.

Another way to evaluate your fees is to be aware of your practice's adjustment rate and compare the variation of each payer. The adjustment rate is the difference between your standard charges and what the payer reimburses for that service. The adjustment rate by specialty is also readily available to use as a comparison. If your practice's adjustment rate falls outside of the norm, this may indicate that the fees are inconsistent with the charging customs of similar providers in the market. Physicians specifically need to understand the difference between contractual and noncontractual adjustments (bad debt, self-pay) and how each affects the ability to collect and the bottom line.

Physicians also need to be aware of price-fixing issues. Physicians from different practices should not discuss or agree on what fees they will charge. However, a practice must evaluate its fees annually against published benchmarks to ensure that its prices are competitive and within the market value.

The physicians must be supportive of all the practice's collection policies, as the staff will mirror the behavior of the physicians. If the physicians do not buy in and endorse the policies the practice develops, the staff may be confused and reluctant to follow any policy or script because it is known that "Doctor X" does not treat his or her patients this way.

It is also important to create collections policies that everyone will endorse. Some of the collections issues that should be addressed include:

- The collection of copayments, deductibles, and coinsurance
- The policy for in- and out-of-network patients

In addition, the answers to the following questions must be agreed upon with all staff members in the practice, including the physicians:

- If a patient shows up without the ability to pay his or her copayment, will the practice see the patient that day?
- If a procedure or service is denied or noncovered, does the patient pay at the time of service or is the patient not seen until he or she is able to pay?
- If a patient owes a balance, will the patient be seen that day?
- If the patient has been turned over to collections, will the practice schedule an appointment or see the patient as a walk-in?

Once the policies are in writing and agreed upon by all the physicians, it is time to train the staff. The practice manager is responsible for training the staff and monitoring the results.

Note

Training on collection policies and procedures should also include speaking in a proper tone of voice and treating people with respect. Looking people in the eye and smiling as you speak will go a long way in achieving positive results. Suggestions for appropriate ways to ask for payment are covered in Chapter 5.

USING PERFORMANCE STANDARDS FOR COLLECTORS

Using performance standards can help you determine how well insurance specialists and/or collectors are performing. These standards should be tied to the practice's monthly collection goals. Usually, the standards relate to the number of days it takes to collect outstanding balances and/or the collection rate of the practice by financial class. To determine the number of days, divide the accounts receivable balance by the average total daily charges. To keep the average charge current, annualize the average daily charges before dividing by 365 days.

REWARDING PERFORMANCE THROUGH BONUS PLANS

Often a practice chooses to reward its staff members for performance that contributes to increased collections and to a more pleasant patient experience. For example, a front office staff member might always greet patients with a smile, or an insurance specialist may have worked out a system for collecting a maximum amount for a special procedure.

Incentives can come in the form of certificates of recognition, gift certificates, promotional items, or cash bonuses. Other examples include:

- a coffee cup with the name of the practice on the side;
- a T-shirt with the practice's logo;
- a gift certificate to a local store or restaurant;
- a "free day off" coupon that can be used for an additional paid vacation day;
- a plant for the employee's desk; or
- a certificate to display on the wall or in the work area.

Keep in mind, however, that these incentives and how these incentives are earned must be clearly defined. Larger incentives may have to comply with accounting restrictions and may have to be reported by employees as income.

APPLYING CODING KNOWLEDGE

Most billing and collections staff members need to have a cursory knowledge of coding, in particular the coding related to the specialty of the practice. This knowledge is critical to understanding appropriate and inappropriate payer claims edits and other payment rationales.

Staff members should be aware of the following basics about coding:

- Current Procedural Terminology (CPT®) and International Classification of Diseases, Ninth Revision (ICD-9) codes are added and deleted each year. They should be updated in the practice's information management system.
- Some CPT codes stand alone and represent the entire procedure.

- Some CPT codes are traditionally bundled with other codes to represent a procedure.
- Some CPT codes require modifiers.
- Some payers have specific guidelines and acceptance levels of modifiers, especially state-mandated programs.
- All CPT codes require documentation.

SUMMARY

During a billing and collections assessment, you have the opportunity to reset your billing and collections operations. This can range from the reevaluation of staff members and their skills to evaluation of the information management system used in the process. The assessment gives you a chance to step back and view the process from a fresh perspective.

chapter 5

Getting Paid by the Patient

Payment from the patient is often the most overlooked area in a practice's collection process. Because of the proliferation of managed care plans, it is easy to forget that not all of the cost will be reimbursed by a third party.

COLLECTING AT THE TIME OF SERVICE

An important goal of the practice should be to collect all patient-responsible payments that are due when a patient comes to the office for an appointment. The best time to collect payments is when the patient arrives at the practice and checks in at the front desk. (The patient's insurance information should also be verified at this time.) Or, if payment is not collected during check in, it should be requested when the patient checks out. Of course, when payment by the patient is not allowed by law or contract, collecting does not apply. However, as many as 90% of patients have some form of payment responsibility at the time services are rendered.

The ability to collect appropriate funds begins with the appointment scheduling protocol. The staff member who schedules appointments should know the practice's policies and should proactively express payment expectations at the time the appointment is scheduled. When questions arise, either during the scheduling process or when patients call in for information, the scheduler must be able to respond appropriately. Telling a new patient that all copayments, deductibles, coinsurance, and past due balances are due at the time of service is appropriate. This establishes the foundation for the collection policy at the outset of the relationship. The successful management of accounts receivable, billing, and collecting is a matter of establishing precedents and implementing policies consistently.

Assume that the patient will be paying the copayment when presenting for the encounter. If the patient objects or expresses resistance, the receptionist should remind the patient about the practice's payment policy:

Receptionist: It is our practice policy to collect copayments, deductibles, coinsurance, and past due balances from patients at the time service is rendered.

Or, in the case of resistance:

Receptionist: Per your contract with your insurance company, all amounts owed by you are due at the time service is rendered.

Having the scheduler and the receptionist state the practice's payment policy will eliminate surprise and embarrassment when the request for payment is made. It is also helpful to post a sign at the front desk, as well. The notice might read:

Effective Immediately

XYX Medical Group, to be compliant with federal law, must collect all copayments and deductibles from all patients, without exception. If your insurance plan calls for you to pay a copayment, deductible, or coinsurance, we must collect that money at the time services are rendered.

The next step is the use of an encounter form (or superbill) for all office procedures. Routing well-designed forms to the staff member completing the check-out process allows for a smooth and efficient payment process. The charge information for the day's services will be easy to calculate and available when the patient is checking out. Depending on the practice's policy, the staff member completing the check-out process can make a statement similar to any of the following:

Staff Member: Your charges for today's visit are $50, Mrs. Jones. How would you like to make payment today?
Staff Member: Your charges for the day are $50, Mrs. Jones. We accept payment by debit cards, major credit cards, personal check, and, of course, cash.
Staff Member: Your charges for the day are $50, Mrs. Jones. Will you be taking care of that by cash, check, or charge?

Just as important, if not more so, than what you say is making eye contact and smiling at the patient when you speak.

These are tactful, professional ways for the staff member to ensure that appropriate balances are collected at the time of service. If, for some reason, the patient indicates an inability to make a payment, the staff member should call the billing manager (or, in a smaller practice, the practice manager). The goal is to resolve the situation before the patient leaves. Typically, the staff member who checks out the patient is not authorized to deviate from procedure and will transfer the discussion and decision to the manager. The manager should take the patient to a private room to discuss payment. The element of authority imposed by the billing or practice manager indicates that nonpayment is unacceptable. At the discretion of the manager, the patient may be allowed to leave without paying, but, preferably, with an agreed-upon plan for payment. In some cases, a fee should be charged if the patient is to be billed.

For sizeable balances insurance plans do not pay or for high deductibles that have not been met, the practice manager or designated staff member can help the patient find an acceptable way to pay for the medical care. For larger balances, many practices are now keeping a copy of the patient's credit card to charge after the explanation of benefits (EOB) is received. Educating the patient on what to expect, both medically and financially, increases the likelihood of collecting. Preauthorized credit card payments and in-house payment plans are suitable methods of collecting payment for services. A sample financial agreement for insurance patients who need to pay their bills over time is shown in Form 5-1.

The long-range goal is to develop the understanding that arrangements for payments must be made in advance of the patient encounter. As with most matters related to credit and collection policy, it is essential to be consistent across the patient base. Consistent patterns of collection inform both the staff and the patients that direct patient payment is important. It's your money—ask for it!

OFFERING DISCOUNTS FOR CASH PAYMENTS

Practices are permitted to give a discount to self-pay patients under some circumstances, but not all. Not all self-pay patients are, in fact, legally considered self-pay patients. Self-pay may be classified as follows:

- Patients who do not have health insurance.
- Patients whose insurance fails to cover all of their expenses and the practice is not on assignment with their payer.
- Patients who pay for health expenses out of their own pocket initially but reimburse themselves from pretax accounts established for this purpose.
- Patients who are receiving noncovered services under their health insurance plan.
- Patients who have preexisting conditions.

F O R M   5-1

Sample Financial Agreement

Patient: _____

Person responsible for payment: _____

Address: _____

City: _____ State: _____ Zip: _____

Home phone: _____ Business phone: _____

Other: _____

Description of services: _____

Fee for services $_____

Estimate of insurance benefits $_____

Estimate of patient portion $_____

Payment plan options: _____

I prefer paying 100% of the patient portion of what the insurance does not cover on the first (____) appointment.

I prefer paying 50% of the patient portion of the first (_____) appointment. The remainder is to be paid within 15 days after the insurance company has paid its portion.

In the event the account should become delinquent for a period of thirty (30) days, I hereby acknowledge that I will be responsible for all the balance, interest, court costs, and/or attorney fees.

I hereby certify that I have read and received a copy of the foregoing disclosure statement this _____day of _____, 2_____.

Signature: _____, Responsible Party

Four federal laws govern discounts for health care services:

- False Claims Act
- Medicare Exclusion Statute
- Antikickback Statute
- Civil Monetary Penalties Law

Routine waivers of deductibles and copayments will violate the False Claims Act, the Antikickback Statute, and the Civil Monetary Penalties Law and cause excessive use of items and services paid for by the Medicare program, which leads to problems with the Medicare Exclusion Statute. But many would argue that none of the federal health benefits programs are at issue in the case of self-pay patients.

The Medicare program will pay only for the "reasonable" cost of health care services. Regulations state that "Medicare payment is based on the lesser of the actual charge or the applicable fee schedule amount."

A provider is subject to exclusion from the Medicare program by submitting claims for charges that are "substantially in excess of [the] usual charges." The Centers for Medicare and Medicaid Services (CMS) offer no definitions of "usual charge" or "substantially in excess." And because these terms are not defined, confusion arises in determining whether discounts are permissible.

It is possible that providing routine discounts to self-pay patients and charging them less than the rate billed or paid by the Medicare program could reduce a provider's "actual charge." If this is the case, then submitting claims to Medicare for an amount greater than the actual charge could violate federal law and lead to a reduction in the provider's reimbursement from Medicare or exclusion from the program.

The Civil Monetary Penalties Law prohibits providers from making remuneration if it is likely to influence the patient's choice of provider. Discounts and waivers of coinsurance and deductibles are only permissible when not done routinely and when a good-faith determination of financial need is made. When a provider can demonstrate evidence of financial need, the provider's actual and usual charge will not be affected.

EXHIBIT 5-1

Sample Professional Courtesy and Other Reductions of Professional Fees

Historically, federal statutory restrictions regarding waiver of copayments, deductibles, and coinsurance applied only to Medicare and Medicaid. However, the Health Insurance and Portability Act of 1996 (HIPAA), also known as the Kennedy-Kassebaum bill, expanded federal fraud and abuse provisions to all federal health plans, such as the Civilian Health and Medical Program of the Uniformed Services (CHAMPUS) and the Federal Employees Health Benefits Plan (FEHBP), not just Medicare and Medicaid; and, now makes it a federal crime to defraud private insurance companies. Violations of the contracts with private insurers are considered criminal fraud under HIPAA and can result in fines and criminal prosecution. It can also result in recoupment of previous payments based on lesser amounts. In addition, the practice may no longer be allowed to participate with that carrier.

Waivers of copayments, deductibles, and coinsurance arguably constitute federal health care fraud if the physician knowingly and willfully attempted to defraud a health care plan or obtain money or property by making false or fraudulent representation to the insurance company. Therefore, if the physician knows that he or she was required to collect a copayment or deductible but only billed the insurance company, the physician has committed health care fraud. Furthermore, by representing the charge to be one amount but only holding the patient accountable for a lower amount (the fee minus the copayment or deductible), the physician is making a false statement regarding the charge or fee of the service. In addition to fines, false statements under HIPAA carry prison terms up to five years for each offense. HIPAA also created penalties for health care fraud including sizeable fines and prison terms.

Even though it is understood that in most situations private insurers and the federal government ban waiving the copayment; however, Medicare has some provisions allowing the copayment to be waived for documented indigency. It is also permissible to discount the entire bill.

The independent Boards of Directors of XYZ Medical Practice and ABC Ambulatory Surgery Center, LLC, collectively agree that every effort should be made to be in total compliance with all federal statutes and insurance contracts. Therefore, the physicians of XYZ Medical Practice shall not offer or provide a discount to any individual except to those who can document financial need.

Courtesy of William R. Pupkis, CMPE, Chief Executive Officer, Capital Region Orthopaedic Group, Albany, NY. Used with permission.

Implement a consistent plan for determining financial need that you can demonstrate to the government and other entities, as follows:

- Develop policies that address the issue of providing discounts based on financial need.
- Spell out what constitutes financial need and how it is determined for all patients.
- Refer to the federal poverty guidelines to help determine financial need.

Develop a written policy that states your practice's policy on waiving of copayments and deductibles and professional courtesy discounts. Exhibit 5-1 is a sample for your reference.

CONFIRMING AND GATHERING COPAYMENTS

One of the challenges facing medical practices today is making sense of varying insurance and managed care plans and associated payment policies, including the amounts of copayments and deductibles for which the patient is responsible. To collect payment from the patient when services are rendered, staff members need to know what each plan calls for, and they should be able to relate that information assertively to the patient at the time of check-in.

Not only does failing to collect payment at time of service hurt the practice initially because of the absence of cash flow, but also billing after the fact is costly. Because it can be difficult to collect a small copayment, the practice may allow such payments to be ignored. Thousands of dollars are involved over the year and the loss of this money directly affects the bottom line by increasing the practice's net collections and net-to-gross charge relationship. Following are steps the practice can take to help establish and maintain patient payment responsibility:

- Maintain an up-to-date reference of the patient's account balance at the check-out station.
- Allow different forms of payment, including credit cards, for the unpaid balance.
- Post a sign at the reception desk that details the policy for collecting copayments. (See the example provided earlier in this chapter.)

It is important to keep a handy reference to each plan's specification in the check-out area. Information about all the plans in which the practice participates should be available. In vertical columns across the page, list each procedure's regular charge, what that plan allows and disallows, and the deductible or copayment for which the patient is responsible.

When not directly indicated on the patient's insurance identification card, one way to gather this information is from the plan's representative or the insurer's Web site. An alternative is to review the EOB from each plan. This summary table should be updated periodically so that the most current amounts are received. Do not assume that the same deductible or copayment exists from year to year. Plans change often, and many times the first thing that changes is the copayment amount. Patients change employers as well, so it is wise to get the information and confirm it in several directions. Front office staff members should check the patients' insurance cards. The copayment amount is listed on them. This is the best way to check because an insurance company can have high and low option plans with various copayment amounts.

With this type of information, the practice's front office staff will have a way to determine what the patient owes and will be expected to pay before leaving the office. Although it is essential to ask for payment, train your staff to handle the requests with ease. The copayment can often be built into the system so that the patient amount due is reflected on the encounter with each visit.

Note

Make very sure your office staff is educated on the difference between deductible, copayment, and coinsurance.

Often, the excuse for not paying the copayment or deductible is, "I didn't bring my checkbook." For this reason, most practices accept credit card or debit card payment. Except in very poor areas, most adults carry at least one major credit card. Accepting credit cards entails a discounting fee, which is paid to the credit card carrier. However, it is minimal and allows for immediate payment and makes paying more convenient for the patient.

In some managed care plans, the contract specifically prohibits collecting deductibles and/or copayments until the plan has paid. (These are different from the copayments required at time of service.) If possible, negotiate this out of the contract. Try to retain in writing that you can request payment due if amount due is confirmed with the payer before the visit from the payer's representative.

If the contract does have this provision, however, obtain advance authorization as a verification of benefits paid for when large amounts are at stake. (When called for benefits, insurers are often known to disclaim at the beginning of every call that this is *not* a guarantee of payment. This payment mechanism is similar to that used by car rental agencies and hotels.) Major credit card companies provide forms for patients to sign in advance. This will authorize credit card charges on receipt of partial insurance payments. Ask the patient what maximum charge limit applies to the card to ensure that an excessive amount will not be charged.

When credit cards are accepted in advance for payments due after treatment, as mentioned earlier in this chapter, the practice should send a zero-balance statement to the patient when the charge is made to the credit card. The statement should show the amount due after the insurance payment and note that this amount was paid by credit card. Sending out a statement showing the payment transaction will minimize the need for patients to call with questions about a payment.

Following are six principles for collecting the self-pay portion from patients before they leave your practice:

- Train your staff about the importance of collecting self-pay amounts.
- Know which patients are self-pay, and ensure that the cashier or exit receptionist handles the collection on check-out.
- Keep a cash fund to make change for $5, $10, and $20 bills. Have a simple system to reconcile and replenish the fund at the end of each day.
- Encourage credit or debit card payment.
- Arrange for automatic credit card charge by using a pre-authorized health care form. The patient can authorize charging copayments, deductibles, coinsurance, and other charges for all visits during the year. Asking your patient to sign the form on the first visit takes care of the collection hassle for the rest of the year (unless the card expires or is cancelled).
- Enforce self pay. If a patient refuses to pay as called for under the contract with the carrier, send a bill with a special notice. This will remind the patient of the requirement to pay and indicate that you will notify the Health Maintenance Organization (HMO) if the patient refuses to pay.

It is also important that all physicians in the practice understand the patient collection procedures and support the process.

RECOGNIZING THE IMPORTANCE OF COPAYMENTS

Copayments are an important source of revenue and have a significant financial effect on the medical practice. Collection of copayments is a fundamental component of managed care. In general, when copayments are not collected, patient utilization increases. Insisting on patient payment helps educate patients to seek medical treatment only when they really need it. Remember, too, that when a patient signs on to a plan, it usually includes an agreement that as a subscriber they will pay copayments. Also, practices that do not collect copayments are violating their contracts with payers who require them.

Although copayments are seemingly small amounts, particularly with HMOs, Medicaid patients, or government employees, collecting them is important. Copayments can range from $3 to $150 at the time of this publication. As a simple example of the significance of collecting copayments, if you see four patients in one hour, a $2 copayment amounts to at least $5,000 a year for a specialist and $10,000 a year for a primary care doctor. To discover the potential effect of copayments in your practice, multiply the number of patients you see each day by the average copayment amount, and then multiply that number by the number of days you practice each year. For example:

$$40 \text{ patients per day} \times \$20 = \$800$$

$$\$800 \times 264 \text{ days per year} = \$211,200$$

In addition, also consider the savings in that the practice does not have the added employee or supply expense of sending out and processing statements.

The best way to collect this money is to get it over the counter when services are provided, either during patient check in or checkout. The cost of sending out statements for copayments is essentially prohibitive and seldom results in collection. Unless there is a large balance, trying to collect small amounts is expensive. Small amounts due are often ignored by the patient. Often, he or she assumes the amount is an error or does not want to be bothered to write a check, mail, or use a stamp for such a small balance.

Note

It is most effective to collect copayments when patients check in for an appointment. Practices that collect at check-out run the risk of the patient leaving without paying their copayment.

COLLECTING FROM HSAs, HRAs, AND OTHER HIGH-DEDUCTIBLE PLANS

Health Savings Accounts (HSAs) were introduced in January 2004 as part of the Medicare Prescription Drug Improvement and Modernization Act. They are tax-free medical savings accounts that must be used with a high-deductible health plan (HDHP). Simply stated, individuals pay for their health care out of their HSA until they have met their deductible. Then, the HDHP takes over.

Minors cannot have their own HSA, but a parent can use their HSA funds for direct dependents' health care expenses. Most of the major health care insurers have begun offering high-deductible policies, usually with benefits resembling their pre-ferred provider organization (PPO) products. The HSA portion is generally administered by a bank or financial institution.

Health Reimbursement Accounts (HRAs) are similar to HSAs, but they are funded solely by an employer and are not portable if the individual changes employers. The Internal Revenue Service designed HRAs in 2002. These plans qualify under Section 213 of the Internal Revenue Code. An HRA is also sometime referred to as a "defined contribution plan." HRAs are typically used with a HDHP, but also can be set up independently.

It is often harder to collect payments from patients who belong to plans or programs with high deductibles. Keeping in mind that there is a generation of patients that have only had to deal with copayments until now will help as collection protocols are established. Using the same approach as a self-pay patient is a good start. Promissory notes and agreements may need to be established, and patient education on your policies regarding these new plans is essential. Patients may also be paying for services utilizing their "debit card" issued by their HSA administrator.

Patients with HSAs, HRAs, and other high-deductible plans will also be taking a bigger part in their health care decision making. Therefore, anticipate more inquiries regarding cost and possible discounts offered. Because the balance due will most likely be larger, you may want this type of patient to meet with the business office in private to establish a realistic and workable payment plan before the patient is seen.

Some contracts require that the patient only pays after the EOB is received. Of course, make every attempt to have this omitted from the contract. If you are unable to do so, speak with the payer

FORM 5-2

Collection Success Analysis

Month of _____

Day	Total Office Visits	Total Subject to Patient Payments	Total Office Visits with Patient Payment Received	% Payable Visits to Total Office Visits	% Payment at Time of Service to Total Subject to Payment	% Goal
Totals						

Month Summary Total Office Visits _____

Total Visits with Payment Due _____ (__%)

Total Visits with Payment Received ____ (__%)

Year-To-Date Summary Total Office Visits _____

Total Visits with Payment Due _____ (__%)

Total Visits with Payment Received ____ (__%)

representative about confirming the deductible met and the patient's payment responsibility before the patient is seen.

ESTABLISHING COLLECTION GOALS

A practical way of ensuring payment at the time of service is by setting practice collection goals. This allows for easy tracking and evaluation of adherence. Recommendations for collection goals are:

- 100% of all copayments and
- 80% of all other types of balances (including Medicare's 20% if the patient does not have supplemental insurance).

Monitor the practice's collection rate on a regular basis, using daily reports to compare the number of copayments and balance bills collected with the number that should have been paid. Form 5-2 will help you perform this analysis.

Once policies are established and adherence becomes part of the daily routine of the practice, you can increase the goals for point-of-service collection, which include copayments, deductibles, and self-pay balances.

Conduct periodic audits to evaluate the effectiveness of the collection policy by analyzing the percentage of copayments and deductibles actually paid (at least partially) while patients are being seen. Following are the typical steps to take to perform such an audit:

1. Select a sample of patient office visits (between 10 and 30 separate days).
2. Tabulate all of the visits in which patient payments at the time of service were applicable. This should include self-pay patients who should have paid in full or in part and patients making copayments and deductibles. Exclude visits in which the practice cannot legally accept payment (eg, Medicaid, workers' compensation, and some managed care plans).
3. Count the number of visits in which patients actually made payments.
4. Divide the number of payments by the number of potential payments to compute the percentage of patients making payments at the time of their visits. The higher the percentage, the more efficient the collection process.

The goal of collecting 100% of all appropriate copayments and 80% of other patient-responsible balances may be aggressive at first, but is attainable.

Often, precedents set by other local practices and by previous providers in the same practice have a bearing on the practice's collection policy. In some communities, the standard is to bill a patient's insurance before attempting to collect from the patient. Even if this process is the established mode in the practice and is expected by patients in the service area, change may be appropriate and necessary. Today's health care environment demands better fiscal management and compliance with contract provisions.

MAKING THE MOST OF BALANCE BILLING

If a patient fails to make complete payment at the time of service, it will be necessary to implement another method to collect the amount due. We recommend handing patients who do not pay at the time of service an itemized copy of charges before they leave the practice along with a stamped return envelope. This not only informs them of their payment responsibility but also clearly communicates that payment will be due soon. If preferred, consider issuing a statement within the next 24 hours.

After third-party payments have been collected, the remaining outstanding balances will be the responsibility of the patient. This adjustment process should be clearly outlined in the practice's contracts with third-party and managed care providers. Therefore, the patient and the practice staff should understand this process from the start. Usually, the final balance will be outstanding at the conclusion of payment by the third-party payer. Balance billing must also be addressed so that the practice receives all monies due.

The following outlines a typical billing and collection scenario:

- The patient copayment is collected at the time of service.
- The practice bills for charges associated with the visit on the CMS-1500 claim form or electronically through a clearinghouse. (CMS-1500 is a standard claim form developed by the Centers for Medicare and Medicaid Services [CMS].)
- Insurance or other third party pays a fee-schedule amount (usually less than the billed amount).
- The payment amount minus the billed amount equals the adjustment amount or the balance due.
- The patient is billed the balance due via a statement.
- If patient payment is not received, the patient is sent a collection letter(s).
- The patient is phoned about his or her balance and payment setup.

Most insurance companies allow patients to assign benefits directly to the health care provider. This does not require an arrangement between the physician and the third-party payer or insurance company. It is preferable to encourage the patients to assign benefits. Doing so will enhance the likelihood of collection with very little risk to the patient. However, it should be pointed out to the patient that the assignment of benefits directly to the physician does not relieve the patient of responsibility for payment. While it assures the physician of collecting the fees that the insurance company is contractually obligated to pay, the ultimate responsibility for payment is the patient's.

Many practices defer sending patient statements until they have ascertained how much the insurance company has paid and therefore how much the patient owes. There are different schools of thought pertaining to this matter. Some practices prefer sending bills before payment has been received by the insurance company to demonstrate that the patient is ultimately responsible for payment. On the other hand, it may alarm a patient to see a large outstanding balance when the insurance company has not yet paid its portion, which is usually the greater amount of the total fee. Also, because many patients realize that their insurance companies have not yet paid, they disregard the bill. Thus, sending bills before receiving insurance payments can be a waste of time and effort and not worth the cost.

The practice therefore must determine the best way to proceed. It is most common to wait to send patient bills until the insurance company has been billed and the resulting residual balance ascertained. If the practice is doing an efficient job of collecting copayments and deductibles up front, balance billing will not be as big an issue.

Regardless of when balance billing takes place, at some point the third-party payer will fulfill its financial obligation to the practice. At that point, the practice must aggressively pursue payment from patients. As a part of the practice's overall collection plan, it must have in place a set of protocols to inform patients of the status of their accounts and of the financial and time obligations once third-party payers have fulfilled their financial obligations in a timely manner. A consistent financial policy must clearly outline the practice's requirements for the patient's ultimate payment responsibility, and the patient and all staff members must be familiar with that policy.

Many times, front office staff members are confused about whether physicians can see and treat certain categories of patients. For example, based on various financial implications, staff members may not know whether physicians will see the following types of patients:

- patients who haven't made payments on their delinquent accounts for a certain period;
- managed care patients who arrive for appointments without primary care referrals;
- patients required to make a copayment at time of service who do not have cash, check, or credit card with them; and

- patients who have services requiring precertification whose precertification is not completed.

Obviously, a consistent plan must be followed, with few exceptions. Physicians may desire to see these patients but, because of the status of these patients, simply cannot. These situations should be handled in a professional, consistent, and confidential manner.

An inconsistent financial policy can cause considerable frustration and even embarrassment for staff members. Ultimately, monies will be lost if there are inconsistencies in the financial policy. If no such policy exists, for example, physicians will treat most patients, and the practice will not be paid for the services it renders.

Practices that send statements on a regular basis (whether before or after third-party payers have remitted their portion) should complete and mail them on a monthly basis. Often, the statements are mailed at the end of the month, so they will arrive early the following month. The hope is that this coincides with the time during which patients pay their other bills. Many practices cycle their billing. For example, a practice may divide patient accounts into four groups and send statements out weekly starting with the first group (eg, group one [A–F] statements are sent out during week one; group two [G–M] are sent out during week two, and so on). In addition, statements are often triggered when activity occurs, such as 30 days since the date of service with no payment, or an insurance or patient payment is posted.

If statements are sent before receipt of insurance reimbursement, a note should clearly indicate the pending insurance payment. If no mention of pending insurance payment is made, patients may pay the balance, creating a credit in their account, or they may be upset because they incorrectly assume that the insurance company has refused payment. It is also good practice to check whether the patient's insurance company has not yet paid. Many patients will proactively phone their insurance companies inquiring about when payment will be made.

Some practices selectively write off a remaining balance without sending the patient an account statement. This should not be done under any circumstance, unless the balance is so small that it would cost more than the amount of payment to send the statement. Another option is to once a year run all statements, including those with smaller balances, with a special message addressing the smaller, but older balance. The routine writing off of copayments and deductibles is illegal, especially for Medicare patients.

Therefore, the practice should always make an effort to collect these balances.

Another aspect of balance billing is applying a finance charge for overdue balances. While this is becoming more prevalent, most medical practices do not apply such charges. In most states, a person must have agreed in writing to pay a finance charge. Moreover, a finance charge often violates provider agreements with insurance companies or other third-party payers. With Medicare, applying a finance charge is a violation because it would increase the amount a physician collected to more than the allowable fee. This is the case whether the practice is a participating or nonparticipating provider. In addition, finance charges may violate managed care arrangements because most such contracts stipulate that the physician cannot collect more than the copayment and deductible from the patient.

Nonetheless, as legal precedents are established and patients begin to accept it, practices should consider applying finance fees to overdue bills. Of course, if they have done an effective job of collecting copayments and deductibles up front (as they should), it would be a moot point.

Recently, many practices have instituted a "rebilling" fee. This fee is for the service of rebilling patients monthly if they have not paid the claim in full. These fees may violate payer contracts so it is important to review them before initiating this fee.

The practice should establish a maximum number of patient statements to be sent. Once the cycle is complete with no or intermittent response from the patient, the practice should turn the account over to a collection agency. The practice should also have a policy concerning whether the patient will be seen again once the account has been turned over for collection.

UNDERSTANDING USURY LAWS AND FINANCE CHARGES

Usury refers to charging and collecting rates of interest beyond the legal limit. States vary on the percentage of interest considered usurious. The standard is usually a flat rate or a rate that is tied to a current market rate. Usury laws apply to credit offered whether it is a one lump sum payment or paid over time. Confer with your attorney or professional, who can furnish information about the maximum percentages allowed in your area.

CHARGING FOR NO SHOWS

Charging patients who do not keep their appointments is always a debated topic, and often seen as a necessity. Each unused appointment time is a loss of income, and more important, lost time during which another patient could have received care. Some specialties, such as OB/GYN or pain clinics, will actually state in the patient agreement that more than two "no shows" is viewed as patient noncompliance and will release the patient to another provider.

There are many ways to communicate your no-show policies as well as software packages available that automatically remind your patients about their appointment. If you plan on charging for no shows, ensure that all patients are notified of your policy and make sure that all reminders are, indeed, occurring.

The next decision is when to charge and how much to charge. While some practices charge the first time a patient fails to show up for a scheduled appointment, some send a warning letter emphasizing the need for the patient to meet his or her appointment, and that there will be no-show charges posted to the patient's account with any further occurrences. A no-show charge ranges from $25 to $100. The encounter form pulled or the printed schedule submitted at the end of each day can be used as a charge sheet. Regardless of the amount, it should be paid in full before the patient is seen again, usually upon check-in at the next visit. (It is usually true that only a handful of patients become "repeat offenders.") When there are extenuating circumstances for missing the appointment, the charge can be reversed.

SUMMARY

It is crucial for a practice to collect all patient-responsible payments directly from the patient, preferably at the time of service. Because the typical balance owed by the patient is considerably less than 50% of the total bill, the sooner this balance can be received, the better.

Most managed care plans require the collection of copayments and deductibles. Generally, they can be collected at any time, though it is preferable to collect them at the time services are rendered. Doing so maximizes cash flow and overall collections as a percent of charges.

Often, practices will have some self-pay patients with little or no insurance coverage. In other cases, specific services may not be covered by insurance. In these instances, the practice should work out a specific payment plan with the patient and collect as much as possible up front. Often, this will coincide with the timing of the services. For example, after elective cosmetic surgeries are completed, postoperative services allow a time frame in which to spread out payments. (Note, however, that all elective cosmetic surgeries are paid for up front.) Nonetheless, the practice should have a definitive payment plan for these patients.

In this era of reduced reimbursements and continuing financial pressures, patient payment of balances is ever more important. Whether collection is a legal or contractual obligation should not matter. What is important is that the collection of copayments, deductibles, and other patient-responsible payments is good business.

chapter 6

Getting Paid by Insurers

A third party usually pays most of the total professional charges generated by a physician's office. This third party may be an insurer, such as a Health Maintenance Organization (HMO), a preferred provider organization (PPO), or an insurance company with a standard indemnity insurance plan. There are many types of private carriers, including health plans that are owned by or affiliated with such health care facilities as hospitals. The other major third-party payer is the United States government, primarily through Medicare or Medicaid. We examine Medicare's payment processes in Chapter 7.

In the United States, most health care insurance is provided by thousands of employers to their employees and dependents. Typically, employers contract with third-party insurers. Usually, a portion of the cost is passed on to employees, with the bulk of the premium being paid by the employer.

Insurance companies do not accept the premise that all claims should be paid as submitted. The health care provider must submit an accurate and timely claim with sufficient documentation to receive payment. Often, this requires special approval or pre-authorization before health care service is provided.

In many instances, third parties require special billing forms, medical procedure and diagnosis coding, electronic claim submission, and contractual relationships. As a result, the medical office must have a sophisticated credit and collection policy for its patients and must adhere to the policy as closely as possible. In addition, it should have consistent billing methods to accommodate the third-party insurer, ensuring that all required information is provided on the claim to ensure reimbursement and to avoid delayed reimbursement.

Frequently, the physician must also know what the insurer considers the appropriate processes and relative values for services being performed. The insurance company must also credential the physician, and this often requires the physician's own personal profile, which includes the physician's home address, medical school, continuing medical education (CME) information, professional references, malpractice carrier information, references, and published works.

Note

When adding a new provider to your practice, be sure to allow at least two months lead time to start the credentialing process so that the services provided are reimbursable.

VERIFYING PATIENT INSURANCE

Verifying patient insurance is crucial, especially when a referral or preauthorization is needed. This process can also be quite time consuming, but is one step that cannot be skipped. It is important to always be looking for ways to streamline the process of insurance verification. State everywhere possible that patients should present their insurance identification card upon every visit. Scan copies of the card for the patient's chart and easy visibility by billing staff.

Most systems allow you to note and track referral authorization numbers, such as how many visits approved, and what may need to be approved along the way. It is also important to confirm where on the claim to place these specific numbers to ensure payment at the first filing.

Patients should also sign a financial agreement, even if just a small paragraph on the encounter form, stating they will pay any balance not paid by their insurance, including workers' compensation. The reason for this is because verification of benefits is not a guarantee of payment by the insurer.

USING THE INTERNET

Due to the extensive time spent on the telephone verifying and obtaining authorizations, many payers are implementing processes in which offices can conduct these tasks via their Web site. These payers are making a concerted effort to educate practices on these procedures, which have proven to be, in most cases, a true time-saver for all involved.

If not already implemented, the practice should contact the payer representative about receiving in-service training for the entire administrative staff. Typically, a few key employees are given passwords to gain access to the secured portions of the payer's Web site. During the in-service training, be sure to ask what other points of the Web site can help with practice procedures now being done by telephone or on paper, such as appeals, prescription approval, claims inquiries, and fee schedule verifications.

Whatever the task or application, continually ask payers for how their Web site can assist your practice with office as well as clinical tasks regarding patients' benefits and coverage.

SUBMITTING A CLEAN CLAIM

Once a patient encounter is complete and checked for coding accuracy, the physician's office is responsible for providing adequate and complete information to enable the third-party insurer to promptly process and pay the claim. A breakdown in the process will delay payment or possibly preclude it.

As a result, the process for submitting a clean claim must be supported by a thorough and fully workable billing process. The process includes the following three phases:

- pre-appointment,
- appointment, and
- post-appointment.

The pre-appointment phase is often the best time to verify patient insurance. If the patient has changed insurance carriers, which happens quite often, then the earlier the better for this to be documented in the practice's information system. That way, additional data can be compiled before the appointment and/or authorization can be obtained from the third-party insurer. There may be a different deductible and copayment, as well as specific areas of authorization and verification of coverage.

During the appointment, four important steps occur:

1. Patient information should again be verified. This entails confirming all demographic information about the patient and getting a copy of the front and back of the patient's insurance card, so that proper documentation and coding can be completed. (This was discussed in Chapter 5.)
2. The physician must properly document the services that were performed. Either the physician or the coding assistant must translate that documentation into correct Current Procedural Terminology (CPT®) codes.

3. The charge capture process must be completed. This usually entails summarizing all codes for each patient encounter and relating them to the practice's fee schedule.
4. The time of service payment (as discussed in Chapter 4) is essential during the appointment phase.

After the appointment is completed, during the post-appointment phase, several processes must take place. These processes are the focus of this chapter. There are ten major initiatives that must be completed properly:

- prebilling,
- coding and entering charges and diagnosis,
- posting of patient payments,
- claims transmission,
- payer follow-up,
- payment posting,
- denial management,
- statement generation,
- collections, and
- retrospective and concurrent review.

Prebilling

The first part of the post-appointment process, which is part of the overall goal of submitting a clean claim, is prebilling. Prebilling protocols should be encompassed within regular coding reviews, periodic account reviews of payments, insurance changes and collection activities, and a claims edit process. In effect, these areas of maintenance should be addressed as a function of the management of accounts receivable.

These areas are often neglected. There may not be a staff member who is responsible for the process, or time is not allotted for appropriate individuals to complete this analysis. Nonetheless, the areas of maintenance must be completed regularly.

The claims edit process is a useful tool. Your practice management system should contain a software package that will complete the "claim-scrubbing" process before the actual claim submission. In addition, your claims processing clearinghouse should have a secondary (higher level) scrubber. These will enhance your practice's ability to submit only clean claims.

Note

The claims scrubber will have no way to determine if the patient name is spelled correctly or the identification numbers are transposed.

Claims transmission

Essentially, there are two ways to process claims. The first is on paper and is mostly a manual process that uses traditional mail. The second, and certainly more preferred, is electronic.

Paper claims submission ensures a slow turnaround and payment (usually 45 days or more). In some cases, these claims are also reflective of secondary filings in which they represent a claim filed with a secondary source of payment (eg, Medigap) or a supplemental payer (eg, a liability carrier). Presently, many paper claims are filed for procedural services in which the operative notes must be matched to the claim and submitted with the claim for reimbursement. This is also true for many surgery services.

Electronic filing is more popular and efficient, and in some instances, a requirement. Medicare now requires all practices to submit claims electronically. Electronic filing can also be used for most governmental reimbursement and with large commercial payers. Typically, a clearinghouse processes the claim after it is submitted electronically by the medical practice. This provides the fastest turnaround for payment. Editing and checking behind the claim is required. Ensure that the clearinghouse is submitting all claims that you have contracted to have submitted. Check the report provided by the clearinghouse of the "suspended claims" and determine why they were not sent. Usually, an "unpaid claims" report can also be run from you practice management system.

Payer follow-up

Constant follow-up with payers is essential. For electronic filings, follow-up usually should be done within 21 days of filing if no payment has been received. For manual or paper filings, follow-up is needed in 45 days. The practice should obtain a report that summarizes the open items by payer. Automatic rebilling should not be completed until or unless some communication has taken place, or the practice has a working knowledge of the account balance and its situation. Of course, the rule is to promptly follow up on claims before they age too much.

Payment posting

When the explanation of benefits (EOB) is received from the insurance company, it should be processed, and payments should be posted accurately to the payer and patient account. This should be done on a daily basis. Feedback should be given to the physicians and nurses in regard to coverage for certain CPT codes from the EOB, as well as the diagnosis selected for the CPT code. Was the service coded correctly? Could it be coded differently? Does the procedure match the diagnosis?

Denial management

Part of follow-up is consistently analyzing claims that have been denied. Your practice management software should have tools to help you with this process. If not, the process will have to be done manually. Denied claims should be summarized by type of payer and analyzed to ascertain why they were denied. This should help avert denial in the future.

Statement generation

Accurate statement generation should follow the submission of a clean claim. Statements should be sent on a regular basis—at least monthly—to both the patient and the third-party insurance company. Statements should be separated by the insurance balance and the patient's responsibility. As balances are delayed or age, follow up on them and include the follow-up as part of the ongoing record keeping. Follow-up can also include such actions as including dunning messages on statements.

Collections

Collection is a unique feature of the accounts receivable management process. It is examined in detail later in this chapter.

Retrospective and concurrent review

Analyze key accounts receivable reports throughout the post-appointment phases. These reports include:

- aging reports,
- days in accounts receivable,
- reports of total denials, and
- other pertinent items of information, such as adjustment percentages and write-offs.

Figure 6–1 is a flowchart summarizing the typical processes for submitting a clean claim. It illustrates the processes for both

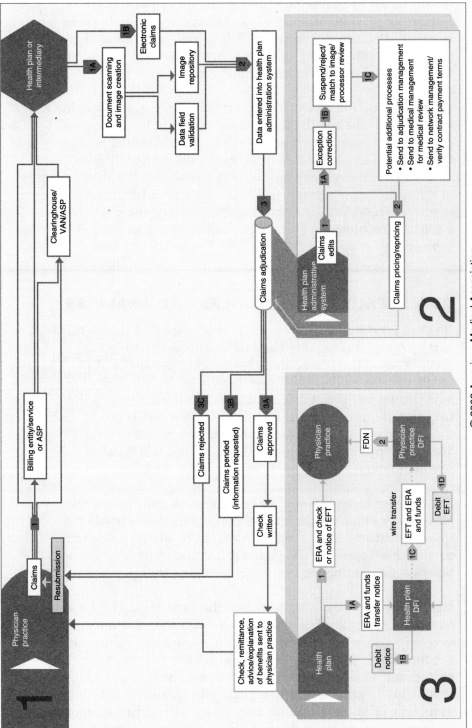

© 2003 American Medical Association

FIGURE 6–1

Claims Processing Flowchart

Note: AMA members may access this flowchart online at the AMA
PSA Web site at www.ama-assn.org/go/psatools.

ASP indicates application service provider; DFI, depository financial institution; EFT, electronic funds transfer; ERA, electronic remittance
advice; FDN, funds deposit notification; VAN, value added network.

manual and electronic filing. Each procedure must be completed for the claim to be paid in a timely and accurate manner. Furthermore, it is important to continuously evaluate these processes to ensure that no breakdowns have occurred. For example, a large number of denials indicates that there is a high likelihood that a malfunction has taken place.

Once the procedures are documented and monitored, specific adherence to the required documentation and form-filing compliance is needed. Often, claims are not accepted because they include incomplete or inaccurate information. Table 6–1 summarizes items that may stand in the way of the submission of clean claims. If a practice continuously monitors these items to ensure that they are handled appropriately, there will be a greater likelihood of clean claim submission and prompt payment.

DEVELOPING PAYER PROFILES AND ANALYSES

It is not good business practice for a physician to ignore third-party payers. In fact, it is essentially impossible to ignore them because they make most health care payments. As a result, physicians and staff members must be familiar with how third-party reimbursement works and what can be done to obtain the most from these payers. If a direct contract with the third party exists, errors in billing will result in a direct loss to the practice. At the very least, errors will result in payment delay.

The credit manager should be familiar with the various third-party payers and should know their requirements better than the patient does. Emphasis should be placed on third parties that represent the greatest number of patients in the practice and distinctive filing requirements that payers may have.

Most third-party insurers have specific agreements that specify how they agree to reimburse physicians. Thus, it is important to develop a summary or profile of each third-party insurer. Profiles should include each payer's contractual requirements for reimbursement, medical payment policies, and its procedural protocols. It is virtually impossible to keep up with this information without some type of automated summary along with periodic reporting. Continually evaluate and update the summary so that it is current. This information will assist both the billing and collection staff. Further, if the summary is up to date, it is more likely that claims will be clean.

TABLE 6-1

Clean Claim Interventions

Assignment	Accept assignment box is checked inappropriately.
Authorization	Claim form did not list the mandatory authorization number or the referral form is missing. Or, the date of service changed and new authorization was not obtained, or the procedure code changed and new authorization was not obtained.
CPT-4	Invalid CPT-4 code was used.
Codes	Invalid revenue codes printed on a UB82 facility claim. Medicaid emergency code, injury code, resources code, other insurance code, and/or Medicare status code is invalid or missing. Invalid insurance codes, ie, 999 (unknown) were input.
Contract Number	Subscriber's contract number is missing or invalid.
Dates	Missing or incorrect dates, such as admission and discharge dates, duplicate dates of service for same procedure code, dates of last menstrual period, first symptom, and so on.
Diagnosis	Diagnosis code is missing or invalid.
Group Number	Missing group number on claim form.
Identification Number	Physician's provider identification or license number is missing on claim form.
Incorrect Balance	Incorrect balance printing on claims. Claims involving coordination of benefits have to be manually adjusted to reflect the correct payment received and amount due.
Insurance Information	Subscriber's name, subscriber's sex, social security number, group, and/or plan number is missing or invalid. Medicare identification cannot have a space or hyphen between the numeric and alpha character. Names must appear exactly as they appear on the patient's identification card.
Modifiers	Missing modifier on a procedure that mandates the usage of one.
Other	Units (quantity) are incorrect and are manually changed or deleted on UB82 claims for Blue Cross facility charges.
Patient Information	Patient's gender missing or invalid, patient's address invalid, birth date is missing, and so on.
Physician Notes	Procedures that always require documentation are not matched with documentation. Documentation is requested from the appropriate source.
Place	Place of service is incorrect.
Primary Sponsor	Medicaid recipients who have a primary sponsor must reflect the primary sponsor's name, identification, and type on professional and/or facility claims.
Private Payer Service Code	Private payer service code is missing or invalid.
Provider	Provider (physician) information is missing or incorrect (eg, provider identification, license number, and so on).
Referral	Referring physician's name and/or identification is missing on claim form.
Type Number	Type of bill incorrect on facility claims. Type of bill varies according to first time claim, status, coordination of benefits, and so on.
Type Service	Type of service is listed incorrectly on claim form.

A payer profile may be completed by an appointed staff person or outsourced by a central processing organization, such as a management services organization, an independent practice association, or some other service organization that can maintain data on an up-to-date basis. Regardless of the means by which the information is maintained, each practice should have a complete and thorough update of its payers' profiles, especially of the most prominent payers. The profiles should be analyzed on a regular basis to ascertain the methodologies, procedures, and overall appropriateness of reimbursement. Forms 6–1 and 6–2 can be used to develop such profiles.

It is best to have a direct relationship with an account representative from the third party. Such a relationship may not only allow easier access to the insurance company, but also may enable a more responsive series of actions, which may ultimately result in a prompter payment.

If these methods prove to be unsuccessful, get more aggressive. Send statement filings, make telephone calls, and contact the state insurance commissioner. Another way to influence payment is to have patients contact the insurance company directly or express concern to their employer, asking the employer to request payment from the insurance company. When the patient is reminded that the balance due is his or her responsibility, this will accelerate the patient's interest in resolving the matter.

Note
When an account is turned over to collections, it should be taken off the account. The patient's account should be flagged that it has been turned over to collections.es.

Every medical practice should use a series of collection letters to obtain payments on delinquent third-party insurer and patient accounts. Ideally, the computer system should generate these letters automatically. Many systems have this excellent collections tool, but often, practices do not use it appropriately or at all. All staff members who have collections responsibilities should learn to use this automated feature.

When possible, the computer system should also automatically generate statements for accounts on which no payments have been made in the last 60, 90, and 120 days. Occasionally, a balance is delinquent because of miscommunication. Statements provide prompt recognition of this outstanding balance owed to the practice.

FORM 6-1

Payer Plan Profiles*

Payer Plan Name and Third-Party Administrator	Employer	Number of Employees	Copayment	Recommended Withhold Percent	Fee Basis	Claims Turn-around Time	Renewal Date Termination Rights	Time Limits on Filing	Hold Harmless Clause	Hospital Providers	Laboratory Providers

* Includes specific managed care plans

71

FORM 6-2

Payer Organization Profiles[*]

Payer	Contact/ Phone	Employer	Fee Structure	Identification Card Description	Copayment	Benefit Exclusions	Hospital	Lab	X ray	Other	Renewal Date	Referral by Physician Plan (Identified by the Practice)

* Includes specific third-party organizations

Successful ways to bill and collect from slow payers include the
following recommendations:

- Develop expertise by payer.
- Have systems in place to identify improper, inaccurate, and
  underpaid remittances.
- Use an automated process to ask for and supply information
  (eg, your standardized monthly reporting).
- Establish performance standards for collectors (eg, dollars
  collected, aging of accounts).
- Establish performance-based incentive pay.
- Require supervisory personnel to follow up on unpaid claims
  aged over 120 days.
- Establish a summary feedback-to-charge source.
- Require (allow) physicians and practice managers to have
  strategic input and operational influence.
- Make certain payers know that if they delay payments, they
  will be aggressively pursued. Speak with a supervisor.
- Review performance of accounts receivable by provider and
  payer. Require collectors to monitor this also.
- Institute and follow a system for addressing unpaid or
  rejected claims.

DEALING WITH SLOW INSURANCE PAYERS

Typically, there is a huge variance in the promptness of payments
by third-party insurers. Some payers are very responsive and pay
within a reasonable time of claim submission.

Include the characteristics and reputation for timeliness of payments in the evaluation of each third-party insurer. Then, when
you evaluate and negotiate managed care contracts, make sure to
consider timeliness. Contact other medical offices or perhaps the
state insurance commission to ascertain the reputation of the
third-party insurer. Often, problems can be averted by early
knowledge of the third parties' reputation.

In addition, consider adding language to the contract to require the
insurance company to pay within a certain number of days from
claim submission. Usually, this is in the 30- to 40-day range, with a
shorter amount of time for electronic claim filing, such as 15 days.

Once the claim has aged, dealing with the slow payer becomes
more problematic. The best solution is to constantly monitor
accounts so that no payer's balances extend beyond a reasonable

period. For example, once an account has reached the 45-day point, the practice should contact the insurance company.

Prompt pay laws

Knowing the prompt pay laws is essential for timely filing as well as in the case of appealing an unpaid claim. Get a copy of the regulations and make sure you understand them—that is, what the law does and does not do. These rules vary from payer to payer. For example, self-insured Employee Retirement Income Security Act of 1974 (ERISA) plans may be exempt, and Medicare and Medicaid managed-care plans are subject to different pay rules. For the most comprehensive information, contact your state department of insurance and share your findings with your physicians.

Note

See Appendix A for information on the prompt pay statutes and regulations in each state. Contact information is also provided.

Also, carefully review payer contracts to ensure they are not at odds with the law. Does the contract define a clean claim in a narrower way than the prompt pay law? Do state laws supersede what is in the contract? Does the contract have amendments tucked way in fine print that either modifies claims requirements or requires physicians to accept a lower interest rate than the laws calls for? Do not automatically accept amendments without thorough legal review.

Note

If you receive interest income from payers, track it separately for accurate income reporting. Otherwise, you will skew your payment profiles.

Recoupment of payments made by payers

Payers "audit" payments made to providers going back several years, then deduct payments (ie, offsets) from current reimbursements to recoup what they deem as overpayment from those claims audited. Many contracts now address this specifically within the language. A typical statement may be as follows: "The payer has the right to go back anywhere from 12 to 36 months regarding previous claims, and any overpayment discovered may be deducted from future payments made to the practice." Another statement may be: "When an overpayment is discovered as a result of a claims audit, the practice will receive a notice of this overpayment and is required to reimburse the payer with 45 days. If the payment is not received, the payer can deduct the amount owed from a future payment." When reviewing and negotiating payer contracts, any recoupment should not exceed 12 months and should not be deducted from future payments.

IDENTIFYING INCORRECT PAYMENTS

The practice staff is responsible for identifying inaccurate, incorrect, or insufficient payments. Begin by consistently reviewing all EOB forms. Most EOB forms indicate what is being paid, but also what services and procedures have been provided and the amount being paid for each patient. The EOB should also state what is not covered and why. Specific action must be taken to cover this if possible and resubmit the claim immediately. If an EOB includes payment that encompasses many patients, there is sufficient individual information to complete an analysis. A practice must have a standard policy of reviewing EOBs without exception.

Once incorrect payments have been identified, staff members must immediately contact the insurance company. It helps if you have already developed rapport with someone—possibly a customer service representative—at the insurance company. Preferably, your contact is a supervisor. If not, a supervisor should be contacted as needed during disputes. The importance of documenting all calls with insurance companies cannot be overemphasized. Documentation should include the name of the representative, date, time, and what was said in the conversation. This documentation will be the basis for any appeals that occur.

To determine whether you need to speak with a supervisor, ask the customer service representative whether he or she would be able to solve your problem if they agree with your position. If the answer is "no," find out who the supervisor is and continue the discussion with that individual. If the answer is "yes," determine whether the customer service representative has true authority to resolve the claim at this point or if the supervisor should nonetheless be contacted.

Although it is rare, some insurance companies require practices to use specific forms for their claims. These companies also create their own procedure codes instead of using CPT codes. This may be especially true with governmental programs. If such an insurance company represents only a small part of the practices' patient base, the practice may decide to terminate the relationship with the insurance company because of its bureaucracy. Usually, the best option is to segregate these claims and have a particular employee learn the system and work the claims as a separate batch.

It is important to have time standards and sequence for collection activities. The process must move along as rapidly as possible and not get bogged down in the daily activities of the regular billing process. If a mistake has resulted in an underpayment, it does not cost the insurance company anything for resolution to be delayed.

We recommend charting the performance of each payer. This should include the total number of incorrect payments versus the total number of claims and the number of days of follow-up and the time expended to collect correct payment. This simple process will help you monitor insurance companies that consistently submit incorrect payments.

Monitoring the outstanding accounts receivable via a thorough and complete aging schedule will also alert the billing manager about accounts that are problematic. Once a payment has been posted, the only difference that should remain is the difference between the gross charge and the agreed-on contractual amount. Some contractual agreements require this balance to be written off. Others allow you to bill the patient for the balance. Often, practices do not write off the difference between their gross and net charges when payments are received. This makes it har to ascertain whether an amount left on an account is a result of underpayment. Thus, it is important to write off these balances at the time of receipt of payment if this is the practice's policy.

AUTOMATING REQUESTS FOR INFORMATION FROM THE PROVIDER

A practice must be able to communicate using automated, interactive processes in order to substantiate its services. Instantaneous communication prevents time lost in the mail system, lost paper, and telephone tag. More and more insurance companies are capable of processing electronically submitted claims. The advantages of electronic submission include:

- faster payment,
- quicker error detection,
- reduced mailing costs,
- reduced clerical labor,
- immediate claim payment or denial response,
- greater integrity provided to the whole billing process, and
- overall significant money savings for the practice.

Many interactive systems are currently available and being developed both by private and hospital-based companies that will assist medical practice providers. The Internet and other e-business mechanisms will be invaluable in the future. Practices that are proactive in learning about what is available in terms of the Internet and other means of electronic communication will likely progress the fastest and have the best operating results.

Commonly, electronic claims are filed through a clearinghouse, which charges a fee. A practice should evaluate the total cost of electronic submission, including the cost of equipment and these access fees. Most practices have concluded that the advantages far outweigh the additional costs.

Many Web sites are directed to both physicians and patients. These health resource sites provide a variety of services, including pharmacy, personal medical records, in-home heart monitoring, and specialists to answer questions. Physicians can also tap into practice management and other services that help run a practice, including interactive communications for claims submission. Personalization is key to these sites. The health content is encoded, indexed, and filtered. In the future, Web sites will better link patients to their physicians.

Some companies offer free Web sites to physicians. These sites allow physicians to access data they need. The next opportunity will be online interaction with patients and third-party providers.

INSTITUTING A FOLLOW-UP SYSTEM FOR UNPAID OR REJECTED CLAIMS

Most practices do not receive all of the third-party reimbursements to which they are entitled. For example, a physician group submits 100 insurance claims. Of those, 10 are returned with denial of benefits, 5 are paid at a lower code and then filed, and another 3 are completely unacknowledged. A thorough billing manager follows up on each denied claim upon receipt of the EOB. This will help back-ups from occurring or keep it at a manageable level. The onus is on the billing department to follow up on these denied claims.

The first step in reducing rejected or denied claims is an efficient patient-intake system. This will significantly reduce the number of claim denials and rejections. This process entails the full continuum of services all the way from the front desk to billing. We examined this earlier in the book; suffice it to say that without an efficient process, the number of claim denials will grow exponentially.

No degree of proficiency in patient intake will eliminate claim denials and rejections. Most practices work the oldest claims first. In some cases, this is not the best approach. Newer denials and rejections are fresher in the minds of staff members, and working them first typically results in quick resolution. It is easier to capture missing information and correct inaccuracies on newer claims, so it takes less time to resubmit the claim with corrective actions, and the return on investment is better.

Strive to be as current as possible with claim resubmissions, and adhere to contractual filing requirements. Older denied claims, particularly those that are problematic, should not be neglected. The goal should be to resubmit every claim only once to obtain appropriate reimbursement. Any deferral of payment from an originally filed claim is costly to the practice, if for no other reason than the time involved in collecting the cash.

Patterns should be observed in the resubmission process and in supposedly erroneous or incompletely collected information. Such problems could be caused by any member of the billing collection function, including the physicians themselves. Document the reasons for the denials and share this information with the physicians and the staff members. Once the reasons for a denial have been determined, staff members should be educated to avoid further errors.

The billing manager has the main responsibility for following up on denied claims. If the billing manager does not do the actual work, he or she should continuously monitor the progress of staff members who are working denied claims. Dealing with denied claims requires extra analysis and work, and most people will procrastinate instead of addressing them. It is also the job of the billing manager to ensure that denied claims are handled on a regular basis. Good strategies include monitoring the number of denied claims and setting goals for the percentage of claims to be filed correctly. Appropriate employee incentives should be developed, possibly with additional compensation once certain percentage thresholds are met. Conversely, when the percentage of claim denials increases, corrective action or withholding incentive pay should be considered.

Another key is the availability and use of monthly reports. If all appropriate monthly reports are completed, there will be information on the number of denied claims. The significance of an unpaid claim in an aging report is the most difficult to interpret because there is no overt message to indicate a problem. Unpaid claims are typically identified when they age more. To discover this promptly, the billing manager must regularly run aging analyses, examine them closely, and then act on the results.

Addressing a rejected claim is perhaps the billing manager's highest priority. A rejected claim means that professional fees will never be paid unless action is taken. Therefore, in a manner of speaking, these are a higher priority than current claims that may be paid without a problem. In addition, denial may be a symptom of a larger billing problem that will cause other claims to be denied. If left unattended, the situation will most probably threaten the financial well-being of the practice.

The billing manager should always be thinking of the implications of denied claims, not only as they relate to retrieving those monies, but also in terms of possible patterns and trends for future outstanding claims. Implications involving other claims must be addressed immediately. There may be a software or filing procedure problem, or denial may be due to relatively minor errors that may not directly relate to the requested monies.

APPEALING DENIED CLAIMS

Faced with the prospect of wasting valuable staff time on aging claims, a practice will often begin sending statements to patients, hoping that they will make payment. While it is likely that the patient will not pay, he or she may assist in addressing the insurance company.

Too many physicians ignore the single most effective action to secure full payment of denied medical claims—filing an appeal. The reason is that many physicians and billing managers do not know how to file an appeal. Others assume they will not be successful because they are unsure which regulatory guidelines to cite in their favor.

USING SOFTWARE TO FILE AN APPEAL

Several good software packages aid in the practice for filing appeals. The better ones provide templates for several different appeal letters that cover the most common claim denial reasons. The system automatically provides case law and state statutes to support particular reconsideration. The cost of such software packages is typically reasonable. The prices at the time of this book's publication ranged from a minimum of $500 to as much as $2,000.

To generate an appeal letter, the following information should be entered in the software program: patient information, insurance account, attending physician(s), medical codes, original claim submission dates, and other related data. Then appropriate regulations or legal precedence are cited from the software databases. They could include:

- verification of insurance coverage, including automated on-screen legal forms for benefits verification and assignment;
- local and federal law regarding coverage exclusion, including preexisting, maternity, newborn, violent crime, and substance abuse denials;
- state law and medical necessity and utilization review procedures, including special rulings on cancer and transplant-related procedures;
- Consolidated Omnibus Budget Reconciliation Act (COBRA) and ERISA coverage termination legislation; and
- time reprocessing and late payment interest regulations for each state.

Additional software support includes a database of government contact information for each state, including the insurance commission and Medicaid offices. In addition, integrated Internet links provide access to online resources such as state legislative databases and national health care organizations.

Therefore, it is more appropriate to file an appeal using this software than to rely on a manual system of appeal letters or asking patients to pursue payment. Patients may have a different definition of medical necessity or other pertinent language than the practice does, and they may blame the practice for making the mistake. Form 6–3 illustrates a sample claims appeal letter.

UNDERSTANDING THE APPEALS PROCESS

The actual appeals process is fairly well defined by managed care organizations, and all managed care organizations have a standard appeal process. Providers and beneficiaries may submit appeals of decisions regarding treatment and reimbursement. If an appeal is necessary, it should be made in writing, outlining the essential course of action. Following are the various levels of appeal:

- urgent review,
- Level 1 appeal,

FORM 6-3

Sample Claim Appeal Letter

To: _____

ATTN: PROVIDER APPEALS DEPT.

Address

City, State, Zip

Re:

Insured/Plan Member: _____

ID number: _____

Group number: _____

Patient name: _____

Claim number: _____

We are appealing your decision and request reconsideration of the attached claim which you denied on _____. We feel these charges should be allowed for the following reason(s):

_____

_____

_____

Thank you for reviewing this claim. Please call if you have any questions at _____.

Sincerely,

- Level 2 appeal, and
- Level 3 appeal.

Urgent review

If authorization is denied for treatment or posttreatment, a provider may request immediate phone consultation with the managed care organization's professional reviewer. Professional reviewers include psychiatrists, psychologists, and physicians. Only physicians may request urgent reviews for medical services. Each third-party payer has a specific protocol of how the appeal is then to proceed.

Level 1 appeal

Generally, the first appeal is made to the reviewer or clerk who initially rejected or disallowed the claim. This appeal involves a review of the records and claims submitted. The reviewer may request the clinical case record from the provider and conduct an additional assessment. The practice should request a quick determination, perhaps as short as 24 hours. It should be pointed out that during this process, the provider is at risk of receiving no authorization of payment of services. An adverse determination at this level entitles the appellant to a Level 2 review.

Level 2 appeal

A Level 2 appeal is usually an appeal to a physician and/or medical director at the managed care organization. It involves a review of the medical records and claims, as well as any additional information supplied by the provider. Some cases may entail a telephone discussion with the provider. Most managed care organizations use a licensed, board-certified physician or licensed nurse, as applicable. An adverse determination at this level entitles the appellant to a Level 3 appeal.

Level 3 appeal

A Level 3 appeal is usually conducted by a board or committee composed of providers specializing in the treatment in question. The board reviews all events that have transpired up to that point, as well as relevant documentation and any other information from the parties. In some cases, the board may meet with a provider to hear the facts and to ask questions. This is highly recommended from the provider's standpoint. The review board usually meets weekly.

An adverse determination at this level is frequently considered the final decision unless the third-party payer and the medical practice have contractually agreed to arbitration or the plan is subject to a self-insured employer that provides an additional level of appeal.

Other stages

If arbitration is a part of the managed care contract, it will be completed by a designated third party. The arbitrator's decision is typically final and binding. Employers that are self-insured and have hired a third party to administer their insurance plans may require an additional level of appeal. Because self-insured companies effectively make their own rules (within statute restrictions), it is easier for them to grant exceptions or to overrule the insurance administrator. They may also be willing to grant an administrative exemption in support of an employee in good standing. From the provider's standpoint, this is acceptable and preferred in order to obtain the ultimate goal, which is payment for services provided.

Whether the appeal process is made via a software program or administered within the practice or as a part of a defined appeals process, it should be completed in a prompt and orderly manner. As with claim denials and rejections, the burden is on the physician for the loss of reimbursement and working capital to support day-to-day operations. Because the claim will not be paid, in part or full, until the appeals process is completed, timing is of the essence.

There is a right and wrong way to submit an appeal. The wrong way is to resubmit a claim without explaining why it should be reconsidered for payment. The right way is to use a format, as illustrated by Form 6–3, or a more sophisticated software program. Attach the original EOB to the appeal letter. No matter which method is used, the practice should learn from the appeal process.

FILING GRIEVANCES WITH THE STATE INSURANCE COMMISSION

Each state has a regulatory body that oversees the insurance industry. Like most governmental agencies, the insurance commission is intended to be a fair and impartial body that serves the public. Therefore, it should be interested in unfair or potentially unlawful actions by the insurance companies.

When a medical practice believes it is a victim of unfair or illegal treatment by an insurance company, it has the right to submit a grievance to the insurance commission. The practice must understand that states only license certain insurance carriers, not all, and certainly not self-insured plans or government payers. The insurance commission is obligated to investigate the matter and possibly require the insurance company to respond and defend itself. Insurance companies are cognizant of this right. Therefore, leverage is available to the medical practice.

Filing a grievance takes time and effort. Generally, it is best to consider filing a grievance only in the case of consistent and/or significant problems in which the ramifications of lower reimbursement are great. The practice should pick its battles with insurance companies and not be overly concerned about minor issues.

The appropriate time to file a grievance is for less than appropriate reimbursement, delays in payment, and other perceived inappropriate actions on the part of the insurance company. Contact the state's insurance commission to ascertain the requirements and protocols for filing the grievance.

SUMMARY

The process of collecting what is rightly due the medical practice from a third-party insurance company or managed care organization involves appropriately implementing all of the procedural processes into billing and collections system functioning. Follow-up and analysis must be regularly executed. Review of aging reports and performance evaluation reports should also be completed on a regular basis.

Dealing with insurance companies can be challenging. They are large and bureaucratic and may try to wield their power and prestige over the relatively small medical practice. They are often difficult to contact, and it is difficult to find a single individual who has the answers to the medical practice's questions. Nevertheless, the medical practice should be consistent and persistent to ensure that matters are resolved.

Some companies are unresponsive to claim inquiries, or take an unreasonably long time to process a claim or forward a payment. If a company is particularly unresponsive, filing a complaint with the state's insurance commission is appropriate. Generally, however, the most effective tactic for dealing with an unresponsive insurer is to involve the patient. This is especially effective if the practice has helped the patient understand that he or she has the ultimate responsibility for payment.

The practice manager or billing manager should routinely review management reports that relate to insurance collection. Reports that are helpful include revenue generated, number of procedures, revenue by insurance company, aging analysis by insurance company, net receipts, contractual adjustments and write-offs, and claim denial rates. Practices that analyze their reports have a much better handle on the situation, and this ultimately results in a more successful collection effort.

It is easy for the process to get out of control. A defined, well-organized, and assertive effort that is consistent in its daily approach, follows all policies, and allows few exceptions is essential. If the practice follows these protocols, it will likely be successful in dealing with third-party insurance companies.

Getting Paid by Medicare

To ensure correct remittance by Medicare, staff members must have a working knowledge of Medicare's guidelines for reimbursement. These guidelines are related not only to commensurate coding but also to facilitate the administrative process of claims review and payment. Medicare claims must be prepared carefully within the parameters required and allowed by Medicare to avoid incorrect billing of procedures, which can constitute fraud in the eyes of the government. Thus, it is important to follow the guidelines set forth by the Centers for Medicare and Medicaid Services (CMS) to prepare a clean claim for which payment is remitted in a timely fashion.

KNOW WHAT WILL AND WILL NOT BE PAID

Create a reference chart that lists services covered by Medicare similar to the chart shown in Table 7-1. This is a good way to ensure that staff members are educated about the breadth of services covered by Medicare. In addition, the chart may help prevent line-item charging for incurred services that are not covered.

Note

Patients should be informed up front that fees for procedures not covered by Medicare will be collected at the time of service or filed with a secondary insurer.

ADVANCE BENEFICIARY NOTICE

The Advance Beneficiary Notice (ABN) is an official Medicare notification that is required to be presented and explained to patients regarding procedures or lab work that may not be covered by Medicare before such work is performed. For example, when a patient presents for lab testing that Medicare may deem not medically necessary, the patient is to be advised that if Medicare does not deem the procedure medically necessary, the patient will be responsible for payment. It is at that point before the test is performed that the patient is to sign the ABN. The ABN is then filed with the lab work. Form 7-1 illustrates a sample universal ABN form.

TABLE 7-1

Sample Chart of Medicare-Covered Services

Medicare Services	Coverage
Medical Expenses: Physician's services; inpatient and outpatient medical and surgical services and supplies; physical, occupational and speech therapy; diagnostic tests and durable medical equipment (wheelchairs, walkers, hospital beds, oxygen)	Coverage[*]
Clinical Laboratory Services: Blood tests, urinalysis, and more	Coverage[*]
Home Health Care: Intermittent skilled care, home health aide services, durable medical equipment and supplies, and other services	Coverage[*]
Outpatient Hospital Services: Services for the diagnosis or treatment of an illness or injury	Coverage[*]
Blood: As an outpatient, or as part of a Part B–covered service	Coverage[*]
X Rays; Speech Language Pathology Services; Artificial Limbs and Eyes; Arm, Leg, Back, Neck Braces; Kidney Dialysis; Kidney Transplants: Under limited circumstances, heart, lung, and liver transplants in a Medicare-approved facility; limited outpatient drugs; emergency care; limited chiropractic care; medical supplies such as ostomy bags, surgical dressings, splints, and casts; breast prostheses (following a mastectomy); ambulance services (limited)	Limited coverage
Preventive Services: Screening mammogram; ophthalmology vision check (covered if diabetic); pap smear and/or pelvic examination (includes breast exam); colorectal cancer screening; fecal occult blood test; flexible sigmoidoscopy; colonoscopy; barium enema; diabetes monitoring; bone mass measurements; vaccinations (flu shot, pneumococcal, Hepatitis B)	Limited coverage

*Covered if deemed "medically necessary."

FORM 7-1

Universal Advance Beneficiary Notice

Date: _____

Center: _____

I understand that my insurance carrier requires a preauthorization for the procedure I am about to receive or my insurance carrier has denied the procedure for a preexisting condition. This procedure MAY NOT be paid by my insurance company. I understand that the charge for this procedure will be my responsibility and I agree to pay. I will be charged the Private Pay rate.

I am electing to have the procedure. Five (5) working days after my procedure by calling [insert telephone number], I can obtain the form needed to file an insurance claim. It will be my responsibility to file this claim. In the event that my insurance pays the claim and [insert medical practice] is a participating provider with that insurance, by providing the Explanation of Benefits I will be refunded the difference, if any, between what I have paid and what my insurance company pays.

Patient name: _____

Patient address: _____

Procedure done: _____

Date: _____

Amount charged: _____

Responsible party signature: _____

Center witness: _____

Date: _____

KEEP UP WITH POLICY CHANGES

Each year Medicare publishes changes to fees and the allowable procedures in the *Federal Register* (www.gpoaccess.gov/fr/index.html). For example, in 1999, Medicare issued the following change regarding the multiprocedural discount:

> We are replacing the current policy that systematically reduces the practice expense relative value units (RVUs) by 50% for certain services with a policy that will generally identify two levels of practice expense RVUs—facility and nonfacility—for each procedure code. The higher nonfacility practice expense RVUs will be used for services performed in a physician's office and for services furnished to a patient in the patient's home, or facility or institution other than a hospital, skilled nursing facility (SNF), or ambulatory surgical center (ASC). The lower facility practice expense RVUs will be used for services furnished to hospital, SNF, and ASC patients. Note: If a physician performs a procedure at an ASC that is not on the ASC list, use the higher nonfacility practice expense RVU.[*]

In addition, Medicare changed its policy on screening mammograms, pap smear interpretations, bone density studies, electrocardiogram (EKG) bundling, and anesthesia conversion factors.

After you have ensured that you are billing for items that are covered services and that the coding is accurate, you must have an ongoing awareness of the practice's reimbursement levels. Medicare sends out a monthly bulletin to providers that updates the medical practice concerning coverage issues. This bulletin should be read and the information provided to physicians and staff members, then filed in a central location as it is almost certain to be referenced at a later date.

As a practice manager or other manager, you should know how Medicare fee schedules are calculated. The formula is as follows:[†]

$$\text{Payment} = ([\text{RVU work} \times \text{GPCI work}] + [\text{RVU practice expense} \times \text{GPCI}] + [\text{RVU malpractice} \times \text{GPCI malpractice}]) \times \text{Conversion Factor}$$

GPCI indicates geographic practice cost indices; RVU, relative value units.

The Medicare fee schedule for your geographic area is updated annually and posted on the CMS Web site at www.cms.hhs.gov/

---

[*]Health Care Financing Administration. *Summary of Medicine Physician Fee Schedule Database Changes for 1999.* Baltimore, Md: Health Care Financing Administration; 1999.
[†]Health Care Financing Administration. Rules and regulations. *Fed. Reg.* Nov. 2, 1999:64(211).

PhysicianFeeSched. Announcements of changes for the upcoming calendar year, are published in the *Federal Register*, usually in November of each year, but this is subject to change. Depending upon your state, you may need to go to your state's Web site for this information. Continue to reference your state's Web site until the fee schedule is finalized for the next year. More information on fee schedules can be found on the American Medical Association Web site under RBRVS: Resource-Based Relative Value Scale at www.amaassn.org/ama/pub/category/2292.html.

SUBMIT A CLEAN CLAIM

The *1997 Documentation Guidelines for Evaluation and Management Services* published by CMS provide a systematic listing of the requirements for accurate evaluation and management coding under Medicare. Each provider should have these guidelines readily available, and each billing office should use them to determine claim viability.

Note

The *Guidelines* are available on the CMS Web site at www.cms.hhs.gov/MLNEdWebGuide/25_EMDOC.asp.

In addition, Medicare provides an instruction form for the use of the CMS-1500 claim form, which is the insurance claim form required by Medicare. If you have not read this document, you should. The CMS-1500 claim form is available in Portable Document Format (pdf) at www.cms.hhs.gov/cmsforms/downloads/CMS1500.pdf. Hard copy forms may be available from intermediaries, carriers, state agencies, local social security offices, or end-stage renal disease networks that service your state. It helps ensure that the claims filed by your practice will never be rejected because of an administrative error.

A clean claim usually consists of the following:

- All fields in the CMS-1500 claim form are completed, where appropriate.
- All International Classification of Diseases: Ninth Revision (ICD-9) codes are accurately derived.
- All Current Procedural Terminology (CPT®) codes represent services rendered that have been adequately documented.

If a claim is returned unpaid, and not easily corrected for refiling, there should be an appeals process in place for the review and investigation of the remittance advice from Medicare. Once review and investigation have taken place, and a refile is allowed, file another claim as soon as possible.

USE THE MEDICARE APPEALS PROCESS

CMS has a four-level appeals process that became effective May 1, 2005. The new process, which combines Part A and Part B, is contained in 42 Code of Federal Regulations, Part 405, subpart I. (See Table 7-2.)

First level of appeal: redetermination

Physicians must submit written redetermination requests to the Medicare carrier within 120 days of receiving notice of initial determination. At level 1, the provider is not required to have a certain dollar amount to make an appeal.

Second level of appeal: reconsideration

Physicians dissatisfied with a carrier's redetermination decision may file a request for reconsideration to be conducted by a qualified independent contractor (QIC). The appeal must be filed within 180 calendar days of receiving notice of the redetermination decision. At level 2, the provider is not required to have a certain dollar amount to make an appeal.

The QIC reconsideration, serving as an on-the-record review, considers evidence and findings on which the initial determination

TABLE 7-2

Medicare Appeals Process

Medicare Claim Appeals Process		
Level 1	Initial Determination ↓ Redetermination	From initial determination, 120 days to file appeal for redetermination
Level 2	Reconsideration	From redetermination, 180 days to file for reconsideration
Level 3	Administrative law judge hearing	From reconsideration, 60 days to file for an administrative law judge hearing
Level 4	Departmental appeals board review	From administrative law judge hearing, 60 days to file before Medicare Appeals Council
Final Level of Appeal	Federal district court	From Medicare Appeals Council review, 60 days to file before federal district court

and redetermination were based, plus any other evidence submitted by the parties or which the QIC obtains on its own.

The QIC's reconsideration must include the findings of a panel of physicians or appropriate health care professionals and base it on clinical experience; the patient's medical records; and the medical, technical, and scientific evidence on record. When the claim involves physician services, the reviewing professional must be a physician, although not necessarily of the same specialty as the physician whose claims have been denied.

In this stage, physicians must submit a full and early presentation of evidence. The reconsideration request must offer evidence and allegations related to the dispute and explain the reasons for the disagreement with the initial determination and redetermination.[‡]

If a provider fails to submit evidence prior to the issuance of the notice of reconsideration, subsequent consideration of the evidence is prohibited. Accordingly, providers may not be permitted to introduce evidence in later stages of the appeals process if they did not do so at the reconsideration stage.

Third level of appeal: administrative law judge

A provider dissatisfied with a reconsideration decision may request an administrative law judge (ALJ) hearing within 60 days after receipt of the QIC's decision and must meet the amount-in-controversy requirement. The final rule requires ALJ hearings to be conducted by video-teleconference if the technology is available; otherwise, it can be conducted in person or by telephone.

Fourth level of appeal:
Medicare Appeals Council review

Under the jurisdiction of the Departmental Appeals Board of the US Department of Health and Human Services (HHS), a Medicare Appeals Council (MAC) review is the fourth appeal level. A MAC review request, which must be filed within 60 days following receipt of the ALJ's decision, must identify and explain the parts of the ALJ action with which the party disagrees. The MAC will limit its review to the issues raised in the written request, unless the request is from an unrepresented beneficiary.

‡Centers for Medicare and Medicaid Services. Electronic Health Care Claims. Available at: www.cms.hhs.gov/ElectronicBillingEDITrans/08_HealthCareClaims.asp#TopOfPage. Accessed Sept. 7, 2006.

The MAC will grant the parties a reasonable opportunity to file briefs or written statements. The MAC will grant a request for an oral argument if the case raises an important question of law, policy, or fact that cannot be readily decided from the written submissions. If the MAC fails to issue a decision or remand the case within the mandatory time, the provider may request that the appeal go to federal district court.

Final level of appeal: federal district court review

A request for judicial review in federal district court may be filed within 60 days of receipt of the MAC's decision. In a federal district court action, the findings of fact by the secretary of HHS are deemed conclusive if supported by substantial evidence.

USE OF MEDICARE ELECTRONIC DATA INTERCHANGE

Use of Electronic Data Interchange (EDI) transactions allows a provider to submit transactions and be paid for claims faster, and accomplish this at a lower cost than what would be incurred for paper or manual transactions. The following information about submitting electronic claims is available on the CMS Web site:

How to Submit Claims

Claims may be electronically submitted to a Medicare carrier, durable medical equipment regional carrier (DMERC), or a fiscal intermediary (FI) from a provider's office using a computer with software that meets electronic filing requirements as established by the HIPAA claim standard and by meeting CMS requirements contained in the provider enrollment and certification category area of this Web site and the EDI Enrollment page in this section of the Web site. Providers that bill FIs are also permitted to submit claims electronically via direct data entry screens.

Providers can purchase software from a vendor, contract with a billing service or clearinghouse that will provide software or programming support, or use HIPAA-compliant free billing software that is supplied by Medicare carriers, DMERCs, and FIs. Medicare contractors are allowed to collect a fee to recoup their costs up to $25 if a provider requests a Medicare contractor to mail an initial disk or update disks for this free software. Medicare contractors also maintain a list on their providers' Web page that contains the names of vendors whose software is currently being used successfully to submit HIPAA-compliant claims to Medicare. This is done for the benefit of providers interested in purchasing electronic billing software for the first time or in changing their current software.

How Electronic Claims Submission Works

The claim is electronically transmitted in data "packets" from the provider's computer modem to the Medicare contractor's modem over a telephone line. Medicare contractors perform a series of edits. The initial edits are to determine if the claims in a batch meet the basic requirements of the HIPAA standard. If errors are detected at this level, the entire batch of claims would be rejected for correction and resubmission. Claims that pass these initial edits, commonly known as front-end edits or pre-edits, are then edited against implementation guide requirements in those HIPAA claim standards. If errors are detected at this level, only the individual claims that included those errors would be rejected for correction and resubmission. Once the first two levels of edits are passed, each claim is edited for compliance with Medicare coverage and payment policy requirements. Edits at this level could result in rejection of individual claims for correction, or denial of individual claims. In each case, the submitter of the batch or of the individual claims is sent a response that indicates the error to be corrected or the reason for the denial. After successful transmission, an acknowledgement report is generated and is either transmitted back to the submitter of each claim, or placed in an electronic mailbox for downloading by that submitter.

Electronic claims must meet the requirements in the following claim implementation guides adopted as national standard under HIPAA:

- Providers billing an FI must comply with the ASC X12N 837 Institutional Guide (004010X096A1).
- Providers billing a Carrier or DMERC (for other than prescription drugs furnished by retail pharmacies) must comply with the ASC X12N 837 Professional Guide (004010X098A1)
- Providers billing a B DMERC for prescription Drugs furnished by a retail pharmacy must comply with the National Council for Prescription Drug Programs (NCPDP) Telecommunications Standard 5.1 and Batch Standard Version 1.1.

For more information please contact your local Carrier, DMERC, FI, or refer to the Medicare Claims Processing Manual (Pub.100-04), Chapter 24.[§]

PAY ATTENTION TO FRAUD: COMPLIANCE SHOULD BE PART OF EVERYDAY BILLING PRACTICES

The prosecution of health care fraud is at an all-time high. Recent legislation has expanded investigators' reach and has increased their power to impose stiff penalties. Investigation and prosecution of health care fraud is also a top priority for the United States Justice Department. This has resulted in an increase in compliance plan development and continuing education in the area of coding.

Physicians are finding themselves increasingly vulnerable. Under the Health Insurance Portability and Accountability Act of 1996 (HIPAA), physicians may be liable for false claims regardless of whether there was intent to defraud. Moreover, upcoding (using an inaccurate code that would result in a higher payment) is now viewed as a false claim. Because keeping up with changes in evaluation and management codes is extremely

---

[§]42 CFR 405.966.

difficult, many physicians regularly and unknowingly commit fraud. Several organizations that have been active in providing physicians with compliance guidance are the American College of Cardiology, American College of Surgeons, American Society of Internal Medicine, American College of Physicians, and American Academy of Family Physicians. The American Medical Association and the Medical Group Management Association publish compliance guidelines.

Compliance is part of a process that starts with claim development and submission, with admission and registration, and continues through patient care, coding, and billing. Because fraud can occur in so many ways, ongoing education for all staff members and physicians is essential.

As a general rule, a provider will be considered without fault if he or she exercised reasonable care in billing for and accepting payment (ie, the provider complied with all pertinent regulations, made full disclosure of all material facts, and, on the basis of the information available, had a reasonable basis for assuming the payment was correct).[**]

SUMMARY

Getting paid by Medicare is probably easier than getting paid by most third-party payers, simply because Medicare publishes its rules. All of the guidelines are readily available in electronic and hard copy formats. In addition, continuing education is available on a consulting basis and in seminar format. If you can set up your billing and collections system to accurately file Medicare claims and use this as your benchmark, you will likely file correct claims with commercial payers.

However, Medicare may provide the lowest reimbursement per procedure for your practice. Nonetheless, use the formula provided in this chapter to determine expected reimbursement. If reimbursement falls outside of the expected range, it is your right to bring this to the third-party payer's attention—and you should.

[**] Medicare Financial Management Manual (CMS Pub.100-06) § 70.3.

chapter 8

Managing Parallel Payment Systems

One of the most difficult aspects of managing a billing and collections system is coordinating parallel payment systems. *Parallel payment systems* are simply those that require a practice to manage both the fee-for-service and the managed or capitated patient.

Whom do I bill, where, and when? The answer to these questions is often fraught with difficulties. Most standard commercial payers accept claim submission via a CMS-1500 claim form or the standard Medicare claim form, and reimburse based on a set fee schedule.

Traditionally, there are only two options regarding payment systems:

- fee-for-service, which is payment for services rendered at an established rate, and
- capitation, where an established amount of reimbursement is paid on a monthly basis and based on the patient's age per member, per month, no matter how many times the patient is seen that month.

Note

Capitation contracts have decreased dramatically over the past five years, and it is not uncommon for a practice to have no capitated contracts.

MANAGE ON THE FRONT END

Create a tool, such as the matrix shown in Table 8-1, for use by the front office staff. It will give staff members the opportunity to assist with the management of payment systems before a claim has been filed. Suggest that staff members refer to the tool at each encounter to be sure that they understand the parameters of the patient's guarantor information.

TABLE 8-1

Sample Front Office Managed Care Matrix

MCO	Copayment, Deductible, Coinsurance, Other	PSO Collection	Physician Participation	Preauthorization Requirements	Participating Facilities	Notes
Blue Cross	Refer to member identification card	$10	All	MRI Ultrasound Surgical	St Johns	CAP–Do not bill fees Referral number required for visit
Humana	Refer to member identification card	20% of encounter total fees	Smith Jones Wilson	MRI Ultrasound Surgical Labor and delivery	St Johns University Hospital	Be sure to copy card (new as of 1/1/07)
Cigna	Refer to member identification card	$12	Smith Jones Wilson (NOT Chin)	All radiology Surgical Labor and delivery	St Johns University Hospital Baptist	Referral number required for visit

MCO indicates managed care organization; PSO, provider-sponsored organization.

MANAGE ON THE BACK END

Update the form you created for the front office staff members for use by the billing and collections staff. The new form should include all information relevant to the paying history and protocols of the payers. This will make the appeals process much easier for staff members. Have the billing and collections staff meet each week to update the tool. Discussion of the week's claim interactions will be a learning experience. Table 8-2 illustrates what the back office tool may look like.

CAPITATION: VERIFYING COVERAGE AND MONITORING UTILIZATION

Most practices are accustomed to creating an itemized bill for their services. In a managed care and capitated environment, the practice may only collect a copayment. Unlike its fee-for-service counterpart, the capitated patient has a managed care plan that is based on prepayment for services rather than prospective payment. In such a capitated environment, it is essential that coverage is current and verified and that accurate copayments are collected.

A capitated patient's plan typically pays a flat or capitated fee to the provider, regardless of whether the patient is ever seen. In the same way, the fee paid only covers a certain allowance of procedures such as office visits. The practice must provide this information to the payer for utilization purposes, rather than for the calculation of an allowable or a patient-responsibility balance.

Many variables must be considered when managing a capitated patient in the practice environment. For example, some prepaid plans require that patients have authorization prior to referral appointments while other plans do not.

Note

The understanding of the complex requirements of the capitated patient often require unique training of front office and clinical staff members.

Although diminishing in number, capitation may still be a part of your billing and collections process. Other agreements may also still include withholds to providers as part of the contract. Withholds are when a certain percentage of your reimbursement is withheld until year end when the risk is evaluated. The withhold is either paid to the provider or held as an expense to the risk.

TABLE 8-2

Sample Back Office Managed Care Matrix

MCO	Copayment, Deductible, Coinsurance, Other	PSO Collection	Physician Participation	Preauthorization Requirements	Participating Facilities	Front Office Notes	Back Office Notes/Common Adjustment
Blue Cross	Refer to member identification card	$10	All	MRI Ultrasound Surgical	St Johns	CAP-Do not bill fees Referral number required for visit	Multiprocedural w/o MRI on same claim
Humana	Refer to member identification card	20% of encounter total fees	Smith Jones Wilson	MRI Ultrasound Surgical Labor and delivery	St Johns University Hospital	Be sure to copy card (new as of 1/1/07)	Second assist w/o provider # Watch for global period cutoff
Cigna	Refer to member identification card	$12	Smith Jones Wilson (NOT Chin)	All radiology Surgical Labor and delivery	St Johns University Hospital Baptist	Referral number required for visit	29909 is discounted below the fee schedule—refile with documentation

MCO indicates managed care organization; PSO, provider-sponsored organization.

Be careful about penalization for over-utilization. Penalties are often taken out of withhold money prior to distribution. Yet, despite this trend, more than 75% of HMOs that paid physicians under capitated arrangements did not penalize physicians for such practices as over-utilization and excessive referrals. Of the HMOs that reimburse physicians through capitation:

- only one in five penalizes physicians for over-utilization of hospitals;
- slightly more than 11% penalize physicians for a violation of prescribing policies; and
- 13% penalize physicians for excessive specialty referrals.[*]

Do your own practice analysis on capitated patients. What is it costing you per patient to see them?

BILLING FOR FEE-FOR-SERVICE CARVE-OUTS

Fee-for-service carve-outs traditionally are involved in contracts in which a provider has negotiated a lesser rate for average evaluation and management services and a higher rate for a specific volume of specialty procedures. Usually only a few scenarios exist for carve-outs[†]:

- **Discounted fee-for-service.** The specialty group negotiates a set of rates lower than billed charges. This makes sense for low-volume, very unpredictable courses of treatment with high complication rates. A carve-out can also be a capitated per-member-per-month payment that provides for certain Current Procedural Terminology (CPT®) codes as "carved out" and a prenegotiated fee paid in addition to the capitated amount. For example, immunizations, and well-woman checkups are frequently "carved out" because they are considered a "wellness" benefit. Other procedures at times can also be negotiated as a carve-out, such as minor surgeries.
- **Case rates.** The specialty provider is paid a flat fee for specific procedures and/or diagnoses for which the group provides special expertise, regardless of volume of services delivered. This is useful for low- and medium-volume and, usually, high-cost

---

[*]Becton, Dickinson & Co. *Report on Physicians in Managed Care.* Franklin Lakes, NJ: Becton, Dickinson & Co.; 1997.
[†]Soroka L. Specialty carve-outs: shifting the risk to medical specialty groups. Available at www.aispub.com/ManagedCareAdvisor.html. Accessed Aug. 2, 2000.

procedures in which the specialty group can accurately project cost and utilization.

- **Capitation.** The specialty group receives a flat per-member-per-month payment for a defined patient population. This makes sense for specialties with high-volume, predictable utilization patterns, costs, and complication rates.

The carve-out theory of specialty services is behind specialty hospitals such as burn centers, cardiology centers, children's hospitals, and cancer centers. The theory is that the unique expertise, specialized equipment, and higher patient volume will make it possible to deliver better patient outcomes and lower cost than at all-purpose medical facilities. In the past, carve-outs have occurred in the areas of mental health and drug treatment.

Regardless of the form of carve-out, it is another possible nuance in billing and collections management. Ensure that physicians and staff members understand the uniqueness of any carve-out arrangement. More than any other risk arrangement, a carve-out shifts the management burden to the practice.

SUMMARY

Parallel payment systems can be easily managed with the correct tools. The process begins with a thorough understanding of the practice's managed care contracts, their requirements, and their corresponding fees. This information can then be translated into a usable tool for the entire staff. Once the participation process has begun, more information can be gathered about the precertification process, the claims payment history, over- and underpayments, adjustments, and so on. All of this becomes valuable information in the management of the system.

If the protocols and tools are in place, management of parallel payment systems is integrated into the overall management of the practice. This is where you want it. You do not want to have a separate system to manage.

The final key to management of the payment systems is ongoing evolution of the tools and protocols. Use the tools and the information they provide to update practice policies and procedures. Make sure that the system is not static—it should evolve as practice evolves.

Prompt Pay Statutes and Regulations

State	Status/Terms of Law	State Contact	Web Site Address
Alabama	Clean claims must be paid within 45 working days; applies to HMOs only. Legislation pending: 30 days for clean, electronic claims; 35 days for clean, paper claims; applies to all health insurance carriers.	Ray Shearer (334) 206-5366 Alabama Department of Public Health	www.aldoi.gov
Alaska	Claims must be paid within 30 days.	Katie Campbell (907) 465-2515 Alaska Division of Insurance	www.commerce.state .ak.us/ins/home.htm
Arizona	Clean claims must be paid within 30 days or interest payments are required (usually about 10%).	Patricia Moore (602) 912-8444 Arizona Department of Insurance	www.azinsurance.gov www.id.state.az.us
Arkansas	Clean, electronic claims must be paid or denied in 30 calendar days, 45 for paper. There is a 12% per annum late penalty.	John Shields (501) 371-2766 Arkansas Department of Insurance	www.state.ar.us/insurance (Go to Insurance Law, select Legal Division, Rules–Final, #43)

State	Status/Terms of Law	State Contact	Web Site Address
California	Claims must be paidwithin 45 workingdays for an HMO, 30 days for ahealth service plan.Interest accrues at 15% per annum.	Rita Ultreraf (800) 400-0815 California HMO Help Center	www.insurance.ca.gov www.hmohelp.ca.gov
Colorado	Claims must be paid in 30 days if submitted electronically, 45 if paper. Penalty is 10% annually.	Michael Gillis (303) 894-7499 Colorado Division of Insurance	www.dora.state.co.us/insurance (Click Colorado Laws on main menu, select Colorado Statutes, then search for statute 10-16-106.5)
Connecticut	Claims must be paid within 45 working days. Interest accrues at 15% per annum.	Cliff Slicer (860) 297-3889 Connecticut Department of Insurance	www.state.ct.us/cid/ newspay.htm
Delaware	Clean claims must be paid in 45 days.	Libby Miller (302) 739-4251 x158 Delaware Department of Insurance	www.state.de.us/inscom
District of Columbia	None at present although a 40-day timeframe has been proposed. Check Web site for updates.	Evette Alexander (202) 442-7780 District of Columbia Department of Insurance	www.disr.dc.gov

State	Status/Terms of Law	State Contact	Web Site Address
Florida	Clean HMO claims must be paid in 35 days, non-HMO in 45 days. Claims where information was requested must be paid in 120 days. Interest penalty is 10% per year.	Consumer Affairs (850) 922-3100 Florida Department of Insurance	http://servicepoint.fldfs.com
Georgia	Claims must be paid within 15 working days. Interest accrues at 18% per annum.	Yvonne Jones (404) 656-2056 Georgia Office of Insurance Commission	www.ganet.org www.gainsurance.org
Hawaii	Clean, paper claims must be paid in 30 days, electronic claims within 15 days. Interest accrues at 15% per annum. Commissioner may impose fines.	Paul Arcena (808) 536-7702 Hawaii Medical Association	www.capitol.hawaii.gov www.hawaii.gov/dca/areas/ins
Idaho	None. Department of Insurance will investigate abusive patterns.	Joan Skroasch (208) 334-4300 Idaho Department of Insurance	www.doi.state.id.us
Illinois	Clean claims must be paid in 30 days. Interest accrues at 9% per annum.	Customer Service (217) 524-4051 Illinois Department of Insurance	www.idfpr.com/DOI/default2.asp
Indiana	Claims must be paid in 45 days.	Cynthia Tompkins (217) 232-2385 Indiana Department of Insurance	www.state.in.us/idoi/ consumer_services/ guideho.html

State	Status/Terms of Law	State Contact	Web Site Address
Kansas	Claims will be paid in 30 days. Interest accrues at a rate of 1% per month.	Steve O'Neil (785) 296-7826 Kansas Department of Insurance	www.accesskansas.org/ legislative/statutes/index .cgi (Enter statute number 40-2442)
Kentucky	Claims must be paid or denied within 30 working days. Interest accrues at 12% per annum when 31–60 days late, 18% when 61–90 days late, and 21% when 91+ days late.	Cindy Dempsey (800) 595-6053 x303 Kentucky Department of Insurance	http://doi.ppr.ky.gov/kentucky
Louisiana	Claims submitted electronically paid within 25 days. Paper claims submitted in 45 days must be paid in 45 days; submitted after 45 days must be paid in 60 days.	Pam Williams (225) 219-4774 Louisiana Department of Insurance	www.ldi.state.la.us
Maine	Clean claims must be paid within 30 days. Interest accrues at 1.5% per month.	Rick Diamond (207) 624-8475 Maine Bureau of Insurance	http://janus.state.me.us/legis/ statutes/24-A/title24- Asec 2436.html
Maryland	Clean claims must be paid within 30 days. Interest accrues at 1.5% (31–60 days late), 2% (61–120 days), and 2.5% (121+ days), respectively.	Joyce Yensen (410) 539-0872 Maryland State Medical Society	http://mlis.state.md.us/1999rs/ billfile/hb0639.htm (Select Bill 639)
Massachusetts	Clean claims must be paid 45 days after receipt. There is an interest penalty of 1.5% per month.	Walter Marcinkus (617) 521-7777 Massachusetts Division of Insurance	www.state.ma.us/doi

State	Status/Terms of Law	State Contact	Web Site Address
Michigan	Claims must be paid in 60 days with an interest penalty of 12% per annum. (Applies only to noncontracted providers.)	Fran Wallas (517) 335-2057 Michigan Department of Insurance	www.michigan.gov/cis/0,1607, 7-154-10555---,00.html
Minnesota	Clean claims must be paid in 30 days. Interest accrues at 1.5% per month if not paid or denied.	Irene Goldman (651) 359-3569 Minnesota Department of Health	www.revisor.leg.state.mn .us/stats/62Q/75.html
Mississippi	Clean claims must be paid within 45 days. Interest accrues at 1.5% per month.	Anne Kelly (601) 359-3569 Mississippi Department of Insurance	www.doi.state.ms.us
Missouri	Pending signature: claims must be acknowledged within 10 days and paid within 45 days. Once requested information is received, claims must be paid or denied in 15 days. Interest accrues at a monthly rate of 1%. After 40 processing days, submitter is entitled to a per-day penalty: the lesser of half the value of the claim or $20 per claim.	Thomas Holloway (573) 636-5151 Missouri State Medical Association	www.house.state.mo.us/ bills01/bilsum01/truly01/ sHB328T.htm

State	Status/Terms of Law	State Contact	Web Site Address
Montana	Clean claims must be paid within 30 days. Interest accrues at 18% per annum.	Bob Durrand (406) 444-5239 Montana Department of Insurance	www.sao.state.mt.us
Nebraska	Claims must be paid or denied within 15 days of affirmation of liability.	Customer Service (402) 471-0888 Nebraska Department of Insurance	www.doi.ne.gov
Nevada	Claims must be paid in 30 days. Penalty interest accrues at rate set forth in Nevada Revised Statute 99.040.	Mary Robinson (702) 687-7651 Nevada Insurance Division	http://doi.state.nv.us
New Hampshire	Clean paper claims must be paid in 45 days, electronic in 15. There is a 1.5% monthly interest penalty.	Collin Mitchell (603) 271-2261 New Hampshire Department of Insurance	www.state.nh.us/insurance
New Jersey	Clean, electronic claims must be paid within 30 days, paper claims within 40 days.	Chenelle McDevitt (609) 633-0660 New Jersey Department of Health	www.state.nj.us/dobi/insmnu.shtml
New Mexico	Clean claims must be paid within 30 days if electronic, 45 days if paper. Interest accrues at 1.5% per month.	Diana Bonal (505) 827-4561 New Mexico Department of Insurance	http://legis.state.nm.us

State	Status/Terms of Law	State Contact	Web Site Address
New York	Claims must be paid with 45 days. Interest accrues at greater of 12% per year or corporate tax rate determined by Commissioner. Fines up to $500 per day may also be imposed.	New York Medical Society	www.ins.state.ny.us
North Carolina	Claims must be paid or denied within 30 days. There is an annual interest penalty of 18%.	Tracy Stevenson (919) 733-2032 North Carolina Department of Insurance	www.ncdoi.com (Select Search NCDOI and enter "Prompt Pay Statutes")
North Dakota	Claims must be paid within 15 days.	North Dakota Insurance Department	www.nd.gov/ndins
Ohio	Proposed changes to Ohio Revised Code Section 3901.38–Senate Bill 4: claims must be paid or denied within 30 days. There is an interest penalty of 18% per annum.	Molly Pordo (614) 644-2658 Ohio Department of Insurance	www.legislature.state.oh.us/ bills.cfm?ID=124_SB_4
Oklahoma	Clean claims must be paid within 45 days. Penalty of 10% of claim as interest for late claims.	Nora House (405) 271-6868 Oklahoma Department of Health	www.oid.state.ok.us www.oscn.net/applications/ oscn/deliverdocument .asp?id=86431&hits=1373 +1372+1362+1361+705+ 512+511+501+500+
Oregon	Clean claims must be paid in 30 days. A 12% interest penalty applies.	Patrick Fitzgerald (503) 947-7270 Oregon Department of Insurance	www.cbs.state.or.us/ external/ins

State	Status/Terms of Law	State Contact	Web Site Address
Pennsylvania	Clean claims must be paid in 45 days.	Pete Salvatore (717) 783-0442 Pennsylvania Insurance Department	www.ins.state.pa.us/ ins/site/default.asp
Rhode Island	Clean claims must be paid in 30 days. A 12% interest per annum penalty applies.	Rollin Bartlett (401) 222-2223 Rhode Island Department of Insurance	www.dbr.state.ri.us/ insurance.html
South Carolina	Group health insurers must pay claims in 60 days.	Ann Bishop (803) 737-6165 South Carolina Department of Insurance	www.doi.sc.gov/Index.aspx
South Dakota	Electronic claims must be paid in 30 days, paper claims in 45.	Randy Moses (605) 773-3563 South Dakota Department of Insurance	www.state.sd.us/drr2/reg/ insurance
Tennessee	Clean electronic claims must be paid within 21 days, paper in 30. Interest accrues at 1% per month.	Everet Seiner (615) 741-2199 Tennessee Department of Insurance	www.state.tn.us/commerce/ insurance/index.html
Texas	Claims must be paid within 45 days (HMOs only). Interest accrues at 18% per annum.	Paula Herwick (512) 322-4266 Texas Department of Insurance	www.tdi.state.tx.us/consumer workshophd1a.html
Utah	Claims must be paid or denied in 30 days. Penalty interest may be applied according to formula.	Karen McKinley (801) 538-3800 Utah Department of Insurance	www.insurance.utah.gov

State	Status/Terms of Law	State Contact	Web Site Address
Vermont	Claims must be paid or denied in 45 days. Interest penalty is 12% per annum.	Nicole Wideman (802) 828-3301 Vermont Department of Insurance	www.bishca.state.vt.us/ InsurDiv/insur_index.htm
Virginia	Clean claims must be paid within 40 days.	Maureen Stinger (804) 786-3591 Virginia Legislative Services	www.wvinsurance.gov
Washington	95% of the monthly volume of clean claims shall be paid in 30 days. 95% of the monthly volume of all claims shall be paid or denied within 60 days.	Janice Laflash (360) 753-4214 Washington Insurance Commission	www.insurance.wa.gov http://apps.leg.wa.gov/wac/ default.aspx?cite= 284-43-321
West Virginia	Claims must be paid in 30 days if electronic, 40 days if paper. Interest and fines may apply. Interest penalty is 10% per annum.	Denna Wildman (304) 558-3386 West Virginia Division of Insurance	www.wvinsurance.gov
Wisconsin	If clean claims are not paid within 30 days, they are subject to a penalty interest rate of 12% per year.	Complaints and Consumer Service (608) 266-3585 Wisconsin Department of Insurance	www.legis.state.wi.us/rsb/ statutes.html
Wyoming	Claims must be paid within 45 days. Penalties and fines may accrue.	Lloyd Wilder (307) 777-7401 Wyoming Department of Insurance	http://legisweb.state.wy.us

Resources

Many worthwhile resources are available for both educational and training purposes for the practice management staff. The following list includes some of the tools referenced in this book.

CLAIMS PROCESSING

Prepare that Claim: Taking an Active Approach to the Claims Management Process.
American Medical Association. Available at:
www.amaassn.org/ama/pub/category/16548.html.
(AMA member-only content.)

Follow that Claim: Claims Submission, Processing, Adjudication, and Payment.
American Medical Association. Available at:
www.amaassn.org/ama/pub/category/16548.html.
(AMA member-only content.)

Appeal that Claim: Taking an Active Approach to the Claims Management Process.
American Medical Association. Available at:
www.amaassn.org/ama/pub/category/16548.html.
(AMA member-only content.)

Helping Your Patients Understand Their Billing and Payment Responsibilities.
American Medical Association. Available at:
www.amaassn.org/ama/pub/category/16548.html.
(AMA member-only content.)

PRACTICE MANAGEMENT

Performance and Practices of Successful Medical Groups: 2006 Report Based on 2005 Data.
Medical Group Management Association.
To order, call 877-ASK-MGMA (877-275-6462) or go to the online catalog at:
www.mgma.com.

Ambulatory Surgery Center Performance Survey: 2004 Report Based on 2003 Data.
Medical Group Management Association.
To order, call 877-ASK-MGMA (877-275-6462) or go to the online catalog at:
www.mgma.com.

BENCHMARKING

2006 National Fee Analyzer. **Ingenix.** To order, go to the online catalog at: www.ingenixoline.com.

A

access. A person's ability to obtain affordable medical care on a timely basis.

accreditation. An evaluative process in which a health care organization undergoes an examination of its operating procedures to determine whether the procedures meet designated criteria as defined by the accrediting body, and to ensure that the organization meets a specified level of quality.

acquisition. The purchase of one organization by another organization.

actuaries. The insurance professionals who perform the mathematical analysis necessary for setting insurance premium rates.

adjusted community rating (ACR). A rating method under which a health plan or managed care organization (MCO) divides its members into classes or groups based on demographic factors, such as geography, family composition, and age, and then charges all members of a class or group the same premium. The plan cannot consider the experience of a class, group, or tier in developing premium rates. Also known as modified community rating or community rating by class.

administrative services only (ASO) contract. The contract between an employer and a third-party administrator.

advance medical services payment agreement. An agreement between the health care provider and the patient for the patient whose insurance company will not pay for a procedure or service. This notice assists the patient in determining whether to have the procedure or service performed and how they prefer to pay for it.

advanced beneficiary notice (ABN). If Medicare will not pay for a procedure or service, the physician or hospital will request that the patient review and sign an advanced beneficiary notice. This notice assists the patient in determining whether to have the procedure or service performed and how they prefer to pay for it.

agent. A person who is authorized by a managed care organization (MCO) or an insurer to act on its behalf to negotiate, sell, and service managed care contracts.

aggregate stop-loss coverage. A type of stop-loss insurance that provides benefits when a group's total claims during a specified period exceed a stated amount.

all products. An "all-products" provision is a clause in a managed care organization (MCO) physician contract that requires, as a condition of participating in any of the MCO products, that the physician participate in all of the MCO products.

ambulatory care facility (ACF). A medical care center that provides a wide range of health care services,

113

including preventive care, acute care, surgery, and outpatient care, in a centralized facility. Also known as a medical clinic or medical center.

AMA Express Reference cards. The AMA Express Reference coding cards are designed to facilitate proper coding by supplying the most common codes per specialty. Express Reference cards allow providers or staff members to easily find a desired code, which can then be referenced in the proper coding book. Express Reference cards are available for Current Procedural Terminology (CPT®) codes, HCPCS, ICD-9-CM codes, and CPT modifiers.

American National Standards Format (ANSI ASCX12N) Transaction Set 837. The format used to file claims electronically or report encounter data (from third-party vendor). The Transaction Set 837 is used to submit professional claims (CMS-1500) and institutional claims (UB92). Coordination of Benefits (COB) is also part of the Transaction Set 837, which provides the ability to transmit primary payer information to the secondary payer.

ancillary services. Auxiliary or supplemental services, such as diagnostic services, home health services, physical therapy, and occupational therapy, used to support diagnosis and treatment of a patient's condition.

annual maximum benefit amount. The maximum dollar amount set by a managed care organization (MCO) that limits the total amount the plan must pay for all health care services provided to a subscriber in a year.

antitrust laws. Legislation designed to protect commerce from unlawful restraint of trade, price discrimination, price fixing, reduced competition, and monopolies. See also *Sherman Antitrust Act*, *Clayton Act*, and *Federal Trade Commission Act*.

Application Service Provider (ASP). A company that supplies software application and/or software-related services over the Internet via a browser. Health plans generally contract with ASPs for their services, though the physician practice may also be charged a per-transaction fee along with a one-time set-up or monthly fee. ASPs allow physician and payers, primarily health plans, to connect via the Internet.

appropriate care. A diagnostic or treatment measure with expected health benefits that exceed its expected health risks by a wide enough margin to justify the measure.

appropriateness review. An analysis of health care services with the goal of reviewing the extent to which necessary care was provided and unnecessary care was avoided.

associate medical director. Manager whose duties are often defined as a subset of the overall duties of the medical director.

at-risk. Term used to describe a provider organization that bears the insurance risk associated with the health care it provides.

autonomy. An ethical principle that, when applied to managed care, states that managed care organizations and their providers have a duty to respect the right of their members to make decisions about the course of their lives.

B

batch file. The aggregation of multiple claims into one data file.

behavioral health care. The provision of mental health and substance abuse services.

beneficence. An ethical principle that, when applied to managed care, states that each member should be treated in a manner that respects his or her own goals and values and that managed care organizations and their providers have a duty to promote the good of the members as a group.

benefit. The amount an insurance plan will pay a physician, group, or hospital, as stated on an insurance policy, toward the cost of the procedure or service to be performed by the physician.

benefit design. The process a managed care organization (MCO) uses to determine which benefits or the level of benefits that will be offered to its members, the degree to which members will be expected to share the costs of such benefits, and how a member can access medical care through the health plan.

bill/invoice/statement. The summary of a medical bill.

billing entity/service. A company that has been contracted to complete and submit health claims for a physician's practice. The billing entity may provide some additional services on behalf of the physician's practice, including verifying physician and physician practice information (on the claims forms) as well as making sure that the necessary fields have been completed (information has been entered in all fields requested by the clearinghouse or health plan).

blended rating. For groups with limited recorded claim experience, a method of forecasting a group's cost of benefits based partly on a managed care organization's (MCO's) manual rates and partly on the group's experience.

brand. A name, number, term, sign, symbol, design, or combination of these elements that an organization uses to identify one or more products.

broker. A salesperson who has obtained a state license to sell and service contracts of multiple health plans or insurers, and who is ordinarily considered to be an agent of the buyer, not the health plan or insurer.

business integration. The unification of one or more separate business (nonclinical) functions into a single function.

C

capitation. A method of paying for health care services on the basis of the number of patients who are covered for specific services over a specified period of time rather than the cost or number of services that are actually provided.

capped fee. See *fee schedule*.

captive agents. Agents that represent only one health plan or insurer.

carve-out. Specialty health service that a managed care organization (MCO) obtains for members by contracting with a company that specializes in that service. See also *carve-out companies*.

carve-out companies. Organizations that have specialized provider networks and are paid on a capitation or other basis for a specific service, such as mental health, chiropractic, or dental. See also *carve-out*.

case management. A process of identifying plan members with special health care needs, developing a health care strategy that meets those needs, and coordinating and monitoring the care, with the ultimate goal of achieving the optimum health care outcome in an efficient and cost-effective manner. Also known as large case management (LCM).

case-mix adjustment. See *risk-adjustment*.

categorically needy individuals. Enrollees in Medicaid programs who meet traditional Medicaid age and income requirements.

certificate of authority (COA). The license issued by a state to a health maintenance organization (HMO) or insurance company that allows it to conduct business in that state.

Children's Health Insurance Program (CHIP). A program, established by the Balanced Budget Act, designed to provide health assistance to uninsured, low-income children either through separate programs or through expanded eligibility under state Medicaid programs.

Civilian Health and Medical Program of the Uniformed Services (CHAMPUS). A program of medical benefits available to inactive military personnel and military spouses, dependents, and beneficiaries through the Military Health Services System of the Department of Defense. See also *TRICARE*.

claim. An itemized statement of health care services and their costs provided by a hospital, physician's office, or other provider facility. Claims are submitted to the insurer or managed care plan by either the plan member or the provider for payment of the costs incurred.

claimant. The person or entity submitting a claim.

claim form. An application for payment of benefits under a health plan.

claims administration. The process of receiving, reviewing, adjudicating, and processing claims.

claims analysts. See *claims examiners*.

claims edits. Claims edits are a set of business rules that have been established by the payer to ensure that specific fields are completed and Current Procedural Terminology (CPT®) codes are paid in accordance with the payer's business design.

claims examiners. Employees in the claims administration department who consider all the information pertinent to a claim and make decisions about the managed care organization's (MCO's) payment of the claim. Also known as claims analysts.

claims investigation. The process of obtaining all the information necessary to determine the appropriate amount to pay on a given claim.

claims management process. The process of managing the preparation, submission, and collection of health care claims by a physician practice.

claims pricing/claims repricing. The process of adjusting payment of a claim to meet the complex contracts and fee schedules of health plans.

claims supervisors. Employees in the claims administration department who oversee the work of several claims examiners.

Clayton Act. A federal act that forbids certain actions believed to lead to monopolies, including (1) charging different prices to different purchasers of the same product without justifying the price difference and (2) giving a distributor the right to sell a product only if the distributor agrees not to sell competitors' products. The Clayton Act applies to insurance companies only to the extent that state laws do not regulate such activities. See also *antitrust laws*.

clean claim. A claim submitted to an insurance carrier for payment that meets the entire standard submission requirements of a health plan and is accepted for adjudication. If a claim is submitted electronically and is covered by the Health Insurance Portability and Accountability Act of 1996 (HIPAA), a clean claim meets all the submission requirements to be in compliance with that Act.

clearinghouse. A private company that provides connectivity between physicians, billing entities, health plans, payers, and other health care partners for transmission and translation of claims information (primarily electronic) into the specific format required by payers. Clearinghouses may contract with or act on behalf of one or a number of payers, or may contract with physician practices for the transmission and/or translation of claims information.

clinical integration. A type of operational integration that enables patients to receive a variety of health services from the same organization or entity, which streamlines administrative processes and increases the potential for the delivery of high-quality health care.

clinical practice guideline. A utilization and quality management mechanism designed to aid providers in making decisions about the most appropriate course of treatment for a specific clinical case.

clinical status. A type of outcome measure that relates to improvement in biological health status.

clinic model. See *consolidated medical group*.

closed access. A provision that specifies that plan members must obtain medical services only from network providers through a primary care physician to receive benefits.

closed formulary. The provision that only those drugs on a preferred list will be covered by a pharmacy benefit management (PBM) plan or a managed care organization (MCO).

closed-panel HMO. A health maintenance organization (HMO) whose physicians are either HMO employees or belong to a group of physicians that contract with the HMO.

closed PHO. A type of physician–hospital organization that typically limits the number of participating specialists by type of specialty.

closed plans. According to the National Association of Insurance Commissioners' (NAIC's) Quality Assessment and Improvement Model Act, managed care plans that require covered persons to use participating providers.

CMS-1500 (formerly HCFA-1500). The universal claim form (with instructions) used by noninstitutional providers and suppliers to bill Medicare Part B for covered services. It is also used for billing some Medicaid covered services and is the claim form accepted by most health plans.

coinsurance. A method of cost-sharing in a health insurance policy that requires a group member to pay a stated percentage of all remaining eligible medical expenses after the deductible amount has been paid. Coinsurance is usually a percentage of the total medical bill.

community rating. A rating method that sets premiums for financing medical care according to the health plan's expected costs of providing medical benefits to the community as a whole rather than to any subgroup within the community. Both low-risk and high-risk classes are factored into community rating, which spreads the expected medical care costs across the entire community.

community rating by class (CRC). The process of determining premium rates in which a managed care organization categorizes its members into classes or groups based on demographic factors, industry characteristics, or experience and charges the same premium to all members of the same class or group. See also *adjusted community rating*.

compensation committee. Committee of the board of directors that sets general compensation guidelines for a managed care plan, sets the CEO's compensation, and approves and issues stock options.

competitive advantage. A factor, such as the ability to demonstrate quality, that helps a managed care organization compete successfully with other managed care organizations (MCOs) for business.

competitive medical plan (CMP). A federal designation that allows a health plan to enter into a Medicare risk contract without having to obtain federal qualification as a health maintenance organization (HMO).

concurrent authorization. Authorization to deliver health care service that is generated at the time the service is rendered.

conflict of interest. For a managed care organization (MCO) board member, a conflict between self-interest and the best interests of the plan.

consolidated medical group. A large single medical practice that operates in one or a few facilities rather than in many independent offices. The single-specialty or multi-specialty practice group may be formed from previously independent practices and is often owned by a parent company or a hospital. Also known as a medical group practice or clinic model.

Consolidated Omnibus Budget Reconciliation Act (COBRA). A federal act that requires each group health plan to allow employees and certain dependents to continue their group coverage for a stated period of time following a qualifying event that causes the loss of group health coverage. Qualifying events include reduced work hours, death or divorce of a covered employee, and termination of employment.

consolidation. A type of merger that occurs when previously separate providers combine to form a new organization with all the original companies being dissolved.

contract management system. An information system that incorporates membership data and reimbursement arrangements, and analyzes transactions according to contract rules. The system may include features such as decision support, modeling and forecasting, cost reporting, and contract compliance tracking.

coordination of benefits. A system to eliminate duplication of benefits when a patient is covered under more than one group plan. Benefits under the two plans usually are limited to no more than 100% of the claim.

copayment or copay. A specified dollar amount that a member must pay out-of-pocket for a specified service at the time the service is rendered.

corporation. A type of organizational structure that is an artificial entity, invisible, intangible, and existing only in contemplation of the law.

covered expenses. Most insurance plans, whether they are fee-for-service, health maintenance organizations (HMOs), or preferred provider organizations (PPOs), do not pay for all services. Some may not pay for prescription drugs. Others may not pay for mental health care. Covered services are those medical procedures the insurer agrees to pay for, as listed in the policy.

credentialing. The process of obtaining, reviewing, and verifying a provider's credentials—the documentation related to licenses, certifications, training, and other qualifications—for the purpose of determining whether the provider meets the managed care organization's (MCO's) pre-established criteria for participation in the network.

credentialing committee. A committee, which may be a subset of the quality management (QM) committee, that oversees the credentialing process.

credibility. A measure of the statistical predictability of a group's experience.

cure provision. A provider contract clause that specifies a time period (usually 60–90 days) for a party that breaches the contract to remedy the problem and avoid termination of the contract.

Current Procedural Terminology (CPT®), Fourth Edition. A systematic listing and coding of procedures and services performed by physicians and other providers. Each procedure or service is identified with a five-digit code. The use of CPT codes simplifies the reporting of services. With this code set, the procedure or service rendered by the physician or other provider is accurately identified.

D

data field validation. Validation of the information in the data field protects the data base from errors, filters bad data, ensures data fields are completed, and stops submission of data with errors to the third-party payer (ie, insurance carriers).

deductible. A flat amount a group member must pay before the insurer will make any benefit payments. In most cases, a new deductible must be satisfied each calendar year.

demand management. The use of strategies designed to reduce the overall demand for and use of health care services, including any benefit offered by a plan that encourages preventive care, wellness, member self-care, and appropriate utilization of health services.

dental health maintenance organization (DHMO). An organization that provides dental services through a network of providers to its members in exchange for some form of prepayment.

dental point of service (dental POS) option. A dental service plan that allows a member to use either a DHMO network dentist or to seek care from a dentist not in the health maintenance organization (HMO) network. Members choose in-network care or out-of-network care at the time they make their dental appointment and usually incur higher out-of-pocket costs for out-of-network care.

dental preferred provider organization (dental PPO). An organization that provides dental care to its members through a network of dentists who offer discounted fees to the plan members.

diagnostic and treatment codes. Special codes that consist of a brief, specific description of each diagnosis or treatment and a number used to identify each diagnosis and treatment.

disease management (DM). A coordinated system of preventive, diagnostic, and therapeutic measures intended to provide cost-effective, quality health care for a patient population who have or are at risk for a specific chronic illness or medical condition. Also known as disease state management.

disease state management. See *disease management*.

drive time. A measure of geographic accessibility determined by how long members in the plan's service area have to drive to reach a primary care provider.

drug cards. See *pharmaceutical cards*.

drug utilization review (DUR). A review program that evaluates whether drugs are being used safely, effectively, and appropriately.

due process clause. A provider contract provision that gives providers that are terminated with cause the right to appeal the termination.

E

835 payment/remittance advice. Also called "X12835 Health Care Claim Payment & Remittance Advice Transaction," it is the standard format for the electronic data interchange of remittance advice data and the electronic transfer of payment for health care services.

early and periodic screening, diagnostic, and treatment (EPSDT) services. Services, including screening, vision, hearing, and dental services, provided under Medicaid to children under age 21 at intervals that meet recognized standards of medical and dental practices and at other intervals as necessary in order to determine the existence of physical or mental illnesses or conditions. Plans offering Medicaid coverage to EPSDT participants must provide any service that is necessary to treat an illness or condition that is identified by screening.

edits. Criteria that, if unmet, will cause an automated claims processing system to "kick out" a claim for further investigation.

electronic data interchange (EDI). EDI is the interchange of structured data according to agreed message standards between computer systems. Electronic exchange of information in the context of pure EDI effectively means without human intervention.

electronic medical record (EMR). Also called electronic health record (EHR). An automated, on-line medical record containing clinical and demographic information about a patient that is available to providers, ancillary service departments, pharmacies, and others involved in patient treatment or care.

employee benefits consultant. A specialist in employee benefits and insurance who is hired by a group buyer to provide advice on a health plan purchase.

Employee Retirement Income Security Act (ERISA). A broad-reaching law that establishes the rights of pension plan participants, standards for the investment of pension plan assets, and requirements for the disclosure of plan provisions and funding.

employer purchasing coalitions. See *purchasing alliances.*

employment-model IDS. An integrated delivery system (IDS) that generally owns or is affiliated with a hospital and establishes or purchases physician practices and retains the physicians as employees.

enterprise scheduling systems. Information systems that control the use of facilities and resources for such organizations as physician groups, hospitals, and staff model health maintenance organizations (HMOs).

Ethics in Patient Referrals Act. A federal act and its amendments, commonly called the Stark laws, that prohibit a physician from referring patients to laboratories, radiology services, diagnostic services, physical therapy services, home health services, pharmacies, occupational therapy services, and suppliers of durable medical equipment in which the physician has a financial interest.

exception correction. Correction of data that was not able to be read by

scanning. Manual input (keying) of data that was kicked out as an exception in the scanning process.

exchange. The act of one party giving something of value to another party and receiving something of value in return.

exclusions. Specific conditions or circumstances for which the policy will provide benefits.

exclusive provider organization (EPO). A health care benefit arrangement that is similar to a preferred provider organization in administration, structure, and operation, but that does not cover out-of-network care.

exclusive remedy doctrine. A rule that states that employees who are injured on the job are entitled to workers' compensation benefits, but they cannot sue their employers for additional amounts.

executive committee. Committee whose purpose is to provide rapid access to decision making and confidential discussions for a managed care organization (MCO) board of directors.

executive director. In a managed care plan, individual responsible for all operational aspects of the plan. All other officers and key managers report to this person, who in turn reports to the board of directors.

experience. The actual cost of providing health care to a group during a given period of coverage.

experience rating. A rating method under which a managed care organization (MCO) analyzes a group's recorded health care costs by type and calculates the group's premium partly or completely according to the group's experience.

expert system. Software that attempts to replicate the process an expert uses to solve a problem in order to arrive at the same decision that an expert would reach.

explanation of benefits (EOB). The EOB may also be called the explanation of medical benefits (EOMB), remittance advice (RA), or provider claim summary. The health plan EOB indicates the services submitted on the claim by the physician and delineates how much of the charged amount for each service was approved, reduced, or denied. The EOB may provide a reason for a particular adjustment. In addition, the EOB delineates how much of the charged amount is applied to the patient's copayment and/or deductible. EOB format, as well as the information presented, varies from payer to payer.

extensible markup language (XML). Extensible markup language was designed to improve the functionality of the Web by providing more flexible and adaptable information identification. It is called "extensible" because it is not a fixed format. It is actually a language for describing other languages, which allows design of customized markup languages for limitless different types of documents.

F

Federal Employee Health Benefits Program (FEHBP). A voluntary health insurance program administered by the Office of Personnel Management (OPM) for federal employees, retirees, and their dependents and survivors.

Federal Trade Commission Act. A federal act that established the Federal Trade Commission (FTC) and gave the FTC power to work with the Department of Justice to enforce the Clayton Act. The primary function of the FTC is to regulate unfair competition and deceptive business practices, which are presented broadly in the Act. As a result, the FTC also pursues violators of the Sherman Antitrust Act. See also *antitrust laws*.

fee allowance. See *fee schedule*.

fee-for-service (FFS) payment system. A system in which the insurer will either reimburse the group member or pay the provider directly for each covered medical expense after the expense has been incurred.

fee maximum. See *fee schedule*.

fee schedule. The fee determined by a managed care organization (MCO) to be acceptable for a procedure or service, which the physician agrees to accept as payment in full. Also known as a fee allowance, fee maximum, or capped fee.

finance committee. Committee of the board of directors whose duty it is to review financial results, approve budgets, set and approve spending authorities, review the annual audit, and review and approve outside funding sources.

finance director. Chief financial officer responsible for the oversight of all financial and accounting operations, such as billing, management information services, enrollment, and underwriting as well as accounting, fiscal reporting, and budget preparation.

formulary. A listing of drugs, classified by therapeutic category or disease class, that are considered preferred therapy for a given managed population and that are to be used by a managed care organization's (MCO's) providers in prescribing medications.

fully funded plan. A health plan under which an insurer or managed care organization (MCO) bears the financial responsibility of guaranteeing claim payments and paying for all incurred covered benefits and administration costs.

functional status. A patient's ability to perform the activities of daily living.

funding vehicle. In a self-funded plan, the account into which the money that an employer and employees would have paid in premiums to an insurer or managed care organization (MCO) is deposited until the money is paid out.

G

generic substitution. The dispensing of a drug that is the generic equivalent of a drug listed on a pharmacy benefit management plan's formulary. In most cases, generic substitution can be performed without physician approval.

geographic accessibility. Health plan accessibility, generally determined by drive time or number of primary care providers in a service area.

Global Fee. A total charge for a specific set of services, such as obstetrical services that encompass prenatal, delivery, and post-natal care. Managed care organizations will often seek contracts with providers that contain set global fees for certain sets of services. Outliers and carve-outs will be those services not included in the global negotiated rates.

grievances. Formal complaints demanding formal resolution by a managed care plan.

group market. A market segment that includes groups of two or more people that enter into a group contract with a managed care organization (MCO) under which the MCO provides health care coverage to the members of the group.

group model HMO. A health maintenance organization (HMO) that contracts with a multi-specialty group of physicians who are employees of the group practice. Also known as a group practice model HMO.

group practice model HMO. See *group model HMO.*

group practice without walls (GPWW). A legal entity that combines multiple independent physician practices under one umbrella organization and performs certain business operations for the member practices or arranges for these operations to be performed. The GPWW may maintain its own facility for business operations or it may hire another company to provide this function.

guaranteed issue. An insurance policy provision under which all eligible persons who apply for insurance coverage and who meet certain conditions are automatically issued an insurance policy.

H

Health Care Common Procedure Coding System (HCPCS). A uniform method for health care providers and medical suppliers to report professional services, procedures, and supplies. HCPCS was developed by the Centers for Medicare and Medicaid Services (CMS) in 1983.

health care quality. The degree to which health services for individuals and populations increase the likelihood of desired health outcomes and are consistent with current professional knowledge.

Health Care Quality Improvement Act (HCQIA). A federal act that exempts hospitals, group practices, and health maintenance organizations (HMOs) from certain antitrust provisions as they apply to credentialing and peer review so long as these entities adhere to due process standards that are outlined in the Act.

Health Care Quality Improvement Program (HCQIP). A program, established by the Balanced Budget Act of 1997, that seeks to improve the quality of care provided to Medicare beneficiaries by requiring Medicare+ Choice coordinated care plans to undergo periodic quality review by a peer review organization.

Health Information Network (HIN). An electronic system that uses telecommunications devices to link various health care entities within a geographic region in order to exchange patient, clinical, and financial information in an effort to reduce costs and practice better medicine.

Health Insurance Portability and Accountability Act (HIPAA). A federal act that protects people who change jobs, are self-employed, or who have pre-existing medical conditions. HIPAA standardizes an approach to the continuation of health care benefits for individuals and members of small group health plans and establishes parity between the benefits extended to these individuals and those benefits offered to employees in large group plans. The act also contains provisions designed to ensure that prospective or current enrollees in a group health plan are not discriminated against based on health status.

health insurance purchasing co-ops (HPCs). See *purchasing alliances*.

health maintenance organization (HMO). A health care system that assumes or shares both the financial risks and the delivery risks associated with providing comprehensive medical services to a voluntarily enrolled population in a particular geographic area, usually in return for a fixed, prepaid fee. The prepaid monthly premium covers the doctor visits, hospital stays, emergency care, surgery, checkups, lab tests, X rays, and therapy that is rendered by HMO-designated doctors and hospitals.

HMO Act. A 1973 federal law that ensured access for health maintenance organizations (HMOs) to the employer-based insurance market.

hold harmless provision. A contract clause that forbids providers from seeking compensation from patients if the health plan fails to compensate the providers because of insolvency or for any other reason.

I

image creation. Creation of a flat file format (print image) for electronic claims processing.

incorporation by reference. The method of making a document a part of a contract by referring to it in the body of the contract.

incurred but not reported (INBR) claims. Refers to a financial accounting of all services that have been performed but, as a result of a short period of time, have not been invoiced or recorded. These are "bills in the pipeline." This is a crucial concept for proactive providers who are beginning to explore arrangements that put them in the role of adjudicating claims—as the result, perhaps, of operating in a subcapitated system. Failure to account for these potential claims could lead to some very bad decisions. Good administrative operations have fairly sophisticated mathematical models to estimate this amount at any given time.

incurred expense. An expense not yet paid.

indemnity plan. A set dollar amount paid by an insurance policy for an insured loss.

indemnity wraparound policy. An out-of-plan product that a health maintenance organization (HMO) offers through an agreement with an insurance company.

independent agents. Agents that represent the products of several health plans or insurers.

independent practice association (IPA). An organization comprised of individual physicians or physicians in small group practices that contracts with managed care organizations (MCOs) on behalf of its member physicians to provide health care services.

individual market. A market segment composed of customers not eligible for Medicare or Medicaid who are covered under an individual contract for health coverage.

individual stop-loss coverage. A type of stop-loss insurance that provides benefits for claims on an individual that exceed a stated amount in a given period. Also known as specific stop-loss coverage.

in-network. A physician that has a contract with the health insurance company to provide health care to the patient. The patient may still be responsible for a copayment, deductible, and/or coinsurance according to their health insurance company benefit plan.

integrated delivery system (IDS). A provider organization that is fully integrated operationally and clinically to provide a full range of health care services, including physician services, hospital services, and ancillary services.

integration. For provider organizations, the unification of two or more previously separate providers under common ownership or control, or the combination of the business operations of two or more providers that were previously carried out separately and independently.

International Classification of Disease-9th Edition-Clinical Modification (ICD-9-CM). The standard diagnosis coding system for health care claims coordinated by the National Centers for Vital and Health Statistics (NCVHS). ICD-9-CM codes assist physicians in transforming verbal descriptions of diseases, injuries, conditions, and certain procedures into numerical destinations (diagnostic coding).

IPA model HMO. A health maintenance organization that contracts with one or more associations of physicians in independent practice who agree to provide medical services to health maintenance organization (HMO) members.

J

joint venture. A type of partial structural integration in which one or more separate organizations combine resources to achieve a stated objective. The participating companies share ownership of the venture and responsibility for its operations, but usually maintain separate ownership and control over their operations outside of the joint venture.

L

large group. A large pool of individuals for which health coverage is provided by the group sponsor. A large group may be defined as more than 250, 500, 1,000, or some other number of members, depending on the managed care organization (MCO).

lifetime maximum benefit amount. The maximum dollar amount set by a managed care organization (MCO) that limits the total amount the plan must pay for all health care services provided to a subscriber in the subscriber's lifetime.

limited policy. A policy that covers only specified accidents or sicknesses.

loss rate. The number and timing of losses that will occur in a given group of insureds while the coverage is in force.

M

mail-order pharmacy programs. Programs that offer drugs ordered and delivered through the mail to plan members at a reduced cost.

major medical expense insurance. A form of health insurance that provides benefits for most medical expenses up to a high maximum benefit. Such contracts may contain internal limits and are usually subject to deductibles and coinsurance.

managed behavioral health organization (MBHO). An organization that provides behavioral health services using managed care techniques.

managed care. The integration of both the financing and delivery of health care within a system that seeks to manage the accessibility, cost, and quality of that care.

managed care organization (MCO). Any entity that utilizes certain concepts or techniques to manage the accessibility, cost, and quality of health care. Also known as a managed care plan.

managed care plan. See *managed care organization*.

managed dental care. Any dental plan offered by an organization that provides a benefit plan that differs from a traditional fee-for-service plan.

managed indemnity plans. Health insurance plans that are administered like traditional indemnity plans but which include managed care "overlays" such as pre-certification and other utilization review techniques.

Management Services Organization (MSO). An organization, owned by a hospital or a group of investors, that provides management and administrative support services to individual physicians or small group practices in order to relieve physicians of nonmedical business functions so that they can concentrate on the clinical aspects of their practice.

manual rating. A rating method under which a health plan uses the plan's average experience with all groups—and sometimes the experience of other health plans—rather than a particular group's experience to calculate the group's premium. A managed care organization (MCO) often lists manual rates in an underwriting or rating manual.

market segmentation. The process of dividing the total market for a product or service into smaller, more manageable subsets or groups of customers.

market segments. Subsets or manageable groups of customers in a total market.

marketing director. Individual responsible for marketing a managed care plan, whose duties include oversight of marketing representatives, advertising, client relations, and enrollment forecasting.

maximum out-of-pocket. The amount of money an insured will pay in a benefit period in addition to regular premium payments. Noncovered expenses are the patients responsibility in addition to out-of-pocket amounts.

McCarran-Ferguson Act. A federal act that placed the primary responsibility for regulating health insurance companies and health maintenance organizations (HMOs) that service private sector (commercial) plan members at the state level.

Medicaid. A jointly funded federal and state program that provides hospital expense and medical expense coverage to the low-income population and certain aged and disabled individuals.

medical advisory committee. Committee whose purpose is to review general medical management issues brought to it by the medical director.

medical center. See *ambulatory care facility*.

medical clinic. See *ambulatory care facility*.

medical director. Manager in a health care organization responsible for provider relations, provider recruiting, quality and utilization management, and medical policy.

medical foundation. A not-for-profit entity, usually created by a hospital or health system, that purchases and manages physician practices.

medical group practice. See *consolidated medical group*.

medical-necessity review. See *prior authorization*.

medical savings account (MSA). A trust that employees of small businesses may establish to pay for out-of-pocket medical expenses.

medical underwriting. The evaluation of health questionnaires submitted by all proposed plan members to determine the insurability of the group.

medically   needy   individuals. Enrollees in Medicaid programs whose income or assets exceed the maximum threshold for certain federal programs.

Medicare. A federal government hospital expense and medical expense insurance plan primarily for elderly and disabled persons. See also *Medicare Part A*, *Medicare Part B*, and *Medicare Part C*.

Medicare Part A. The part of Medicare that provides basic hospital insurance coverage automatically for most eligible persons. See also *Medicare*.

Medicare Part B. A voluntary program that is part of Medicare and provides benefits to cover the costs of physicians' services. See also *Medicare*.

Medicare Part C. The part of Medicare that expands the list of different types of entities allowed to offer health plans to Medicare beneficiaries. Also known as Medicare+Choice. See also *Medicare*.

Medicare Part D. A voluntary program that is a part of Medicare that provides prescription drug coverage to Medicare beneficiaries.

Medicare+Choice. See *Medicare Part C*.

Medicare+Choice MSAs. Accounts created by contributions from HCFA to pay out-of-pocket medical expenses for Medicare beneficiaries. The accounts are used in conjunction with high-deductible, catastrophic health care policies.

Medicare's National Correct Coding Initiative. The CMS developed the National Correct Coding Initiative (CCI) to promote national correct coding methodologies and to eliminate improper coding. CCI edits are developed based on coding conventions defined in the American Medical Association's *Current Procedural Terminology (CPT®)* codebook, current standards of medical and surgical coding practice, input from national medical specialty societies, and analysis of current coding practice.

Medicare supplement. A private medical expense insurance plan that supplements Medicare coverage. Also known as a Medigap policy.

Medigap policy. See *Medicare supplement*.

member services. The department responsible for helping members with any problems, handling member grievances and complaints, tracking and reporting patterns of problems encountered, and enhancing the relationship between members of the plan and the plan itself.

Mental Health Parity Act (MHPA). A federal act that prohibits group health plans that offer mental health benefits from applying more restrictive limits on coverage for mental illness than for physical illness.

merger. A type of structural integration that occurs when two or more separate providers are legally joined.

messenger model. A type of independent practice association (IPA) that simply negotiates contract terms with managed care organizations (MCOs) on behalf of member physicians, who then contract directly with MCOs using the terms negotiated by the IPA. This type of IPA is most often used with fee-for-service or discounted fee-for-service compensation arrangements.

modified community rating. See *adjusted community rating*.

monthly operating report (MOR). A document that reports the month- and year-to-date financial status of a managed care plan.

N

national accounts. Large group accounts that have employees in more than one geographic area that are covered through a single national contract for health coverage. Contrast with large local groups.

National Practitioner Data Bank (NPDB). A database maintained by the federal government that contains information on physicians and other medical practitioners against whom medical malpractice claims have been settled or other disciplinary actions have been taken.

national standard formats (NSF). Electronic data interchange (EDI) standards that define the techniques for structuring data into the electronic message equivalents of paper-based documents.

network. The group of physicians, hospitals, and other medical care providers that a specific managed care plan has contracted with to deliver medical services to its members.

network model HMO. A health maintenance organization (HMO) that contracts with more than one group practice of physicians or specialty groups.

Newborns' and Mothers' Health Protection Act (NMHPA). A federal law that mandates that coverage for hospital stays for childbirth cannot generally be less than 48 hours for normal deliveries or 96 hours for cesarean births.

no balance billing provision. A provider contract clause that states that the provider agrees to accept the amount the plan pays for medical services as payment in full and not to bill plan members for additional amounts (except for copayments, coinsurance, and deductibles).

noncancelable policy. A policy that guarantees insurance as long as the premium is paid. It is also called a guaranteed renewable policy.

noncovered charges. Costs for medical treatment that a health insurance company does not pay. Determination if treatment is covered by the health insurance policy can be determined before the charges are billed by the physician's office.

nongroup market. A market segment that consists of customers who are covered under an individual contract for health coverage or enrolled in a government program.

non-malfeasance. An ethical principle that, when applied to managed care, states that managed care organizations and their providers are obligated not to harm their members.

o

Omnibus Budget Reconciliation Act (OBRA) of 1990. A federal act that established the Medicare SELECT program, a Medicare supplement that uses a preferred provider organization to supplement Medicare Part B coverage.

open access. A provision that specifies that plan members may self-refer to a specialist, either in-network or out-of-network, at full benefit or at a reduced benefit, without first obtaining a referral from a primary care provider.

open formulary. The provision that drugs on the preferred list and those not on the preferred list will both be covered by a pharmacy benefit management (PBM) plan or managed care organization (MCO).

open-panel HMO. A health maintenance organization (HMO) in which any physician who meets the HMO's standards of care may contract with the HMO as a provider. These physicians typically operate out of their own offices and see other patients as well as HMO members.

open PHO. A type of physician–hospital organization that is available to all of a hospital's eligible medical staff.

operational integration. The consolidation into a single operation or operations that were previously carried out separately by different providers.

operations director. Individual who typically oversees claims, management information services, enrollment, underwriting, member services, and office management.

outcomes measures. Health care quality indicators that gauge the extent to which health care services succeed in improving patient health.

out-of-network. A physician that is not contracted with the patient's health insurance company to provide medical treatment to that patient. The patient is responsible for the payment of the medical care. The physician may agree to submit the medical bill directly to the payer for payment. However, the patient may be responsible for an increased copayment, deductible, coinsurance, and/or additional charges according to their insurance company benefit plan.

out-of-pocket maximums. Dollar amounts set by managed care organizations (MCOs) that limit the amount a member has to pay out of his or her own pocket for particular health care services during a particular time period.

outpatient care. Treatment that is provided to a patient who is able to return home after care without an overnight stay in a hospital or other inpatient facility.

P

parent company. A company that owns another company.

Patient Bill of Rights. Refers to the Consumer Bill of Rights and Responsibilities, a report prepared by the President's Advisory Commission on Consumer Protection and Quality in the Health Care Industry in an effort to ensure the security of patient information, promote health care quality, and improve the availability of health care treatment and services. The report lists a number "rights," subdivided into eight general areas, that all health care consumers should be guaranteed and describes responsibilities that consumers need to accept for the sake of their own health.

patient perception. A type of outcomes measure related to how the patient feels after treatment.

peer review. The analysis of a clinician's care by a group of that clinician's professional colleagues. The provider's care is generally compared to applicable standards of care, and the group's analysis is used as a learning tool for the members of the group.

peer review organizations (PROs). According to the Balanced Budget Act of 1997, organizations or groups of practicing physicians and other health care professionals paid by the federal government to review and evaluate the services provided by other practitioners and to monitor the quality of care given to Medicare patients.

pended. A claims term that refers to a situation in which it is not known whether an authorization has or will be issued for delivery of a health care service, and the case has been set aside for review.

performance measures. Quantitative measures of the quality of care provided by a health plan or provider that consumers, payers, regulators, and others can use to compare the plan or provider to other plans and providers.

personal care physician. See *primary care provider*.

personal care provider. See *primary care provider*.

pharmaceutical cards. Identification cards issued by a pharmacy benefit management plan to plan members. These cards assist pharmacy benefit management (PBM) plans in processing and tracking pharmaceutical claims. Also known as drug cards or prescription cards.

pharmacy and therapeutics committee. Committee charged with developing a formulary, reviewing changes to that formulary, and reviewing abnormal prescription utilization patterns by providers.

pharmacy benefit management (PBM) plan. A type of managed care specialty service organization that seeks to contain the costs, while promoting safer and more efficient use, of prescription drugs or pharmaceuticals. Also known as a prescription benefit management plan.

physician–hospital organization (PHO). A joint venture between a hospital and many or all of its admitting physicians whose primary purpose is contract negotiations with managed care organizations (MCOs) and marketing.

Physician Practice Management (PPM) company. A company, owned by a group of investors, that purchases physicians' practice assets, provides practice management services, and, in most cases, gives physicians a long-term contract to continue working in their practice and sometimes an equity (ownership) position in the company.

physician profiling. In the context of a pharmacy benefit plan, the process of compiling data on physician prescribing patterns and comparing physicians' actual prescribing patterns to expected patterns within select drug categories. Also known as profiling.

plan funding. The method that an employer or other payer or purchaser uses to pay medical benefit costs and administrative expenses.

point-of-service (POS) product. A health care option that allows members to choose at the time medical services are needed whether they will go to a provider within the plan's network or seek medical care outside the network.

pooling. The practice of underwriting a number of small groups as if they constituted one large group.

practice guideline. See *clinical practice guideline*.

pre-authorization. A prospective process to verify coverage of proposed care, and to establish covered length of stay.

pre-certification. A utilization management program that requires the member or the physician to notify the health plan prior to a hospitalization, diagnostic test, or surgical procedure. The notification allows the health plan to provide an authorization number. See also *prospective authorization*.

pre-determination. A health plan requirement that a physician practice must request confirmation from the health plan. In some cases, this confirmation must be in writing, ensuring that a service or procedure to be performed by the physician or health care provider is contained in the patient's benefit coverage.

pre-existing condition. In group health insurance, generally a condition for which an individual received medical care during the three months immediately prior to the effective date of coverage.

preferred provider arrangement (PPA). As defined in state laws, a contract between a health care insurer and a health care provider or group of providers who agree to provide services to persons covered under the contract. Examples include preferred provider organizations (PPOs) and exclusive provider organizations (EPOs).

preferred provider organization (PPO). A health care benefit arrangement designed to supply services at a discounted cost by providing incentives for members to use designated health care providers (who contract with the PPO at a discount), but which also provides coverage for services rendered by health care providers who are not part of the PPO network.

premium. A prepaid payment or series of payments made to a health plan by purchasers, and often plan members, for medical benefits.

premium taxes. State income taxes levied on an insurer's premium income.

prepaid care. Health care services provided to a health maintenance organization (HMO) member in exchange for a fixed, monthly premium paid in advance of the delivery of medical care.

prepaid group practices. Term originally used to describe health care systems that later became known as health maintenance organizations.

prescription benefit management plan. See *pharmacy benefit management plan.*

prescription cards. See *pharmaceutical cards.*

primary care. General medical care that is provided directly to a patient without referral from another physician. It is focused on preventative care and the treatment of routine injuries and illnesses.

primary care case manager (PCCM). In states that have obtained a Section 1915(b) waiver, a primary care provider who contracts directly with the state to provide case management services, such as coordination and delivery of services, to Medicaid patients in an effort to reduce emergency room use, increase preventive care, and improve overall effectiveness by fostering a close physician–patient relationship.

primary care physician. See *primary care provider.*

primary care provider (PCP). A physician or other medical professional who serves as a group member's first contact with a plan's health care system. Also known as a primary care physician, personal care physician, or personal care provider.

primary health insurance company. The health insurance company that is responsible to pay the patient's benefits first when a patient has more than one health insurance plan.

primary source verification. A process through which an organization validates credentialing information from the organization that originally conferred or issued the credentialing element to the practitioner.

print image or electronic flat file format. Flat files are electronic files that contain machine-readable data that is typically encoded as printable characters (print image). A flat file usually contains a series of records (or lines), in which each record is a sequence of fields. A field contains a specific piece of data (eg, an account number).

prior authorization. In the context of a pharmacy benefit management (PBM) plan, a program that requires physicians to obtain certification of medical necessity prior to drug dispensing. Also known as a medical-necessity review.

process measures. Health care quality indicators related to the methods and procedures that a managed care organization and its providers use to furnish care.

profiling. See *physician profiling*.

promise keeping/truth telling. An ethical principle that, when applied to managed care, states that managed care organizations and their providers have a duty to present information honestly and are obligated to honor commitments.

prospective authorization. Authorization to deliver health care service that is issued before any service is rendered. Also known as pre-certification.

provider. Any person (doctor, nurse, dentist) or institution (hospital or clinic) that provides medical care.

Provider Manual. A document that contains information concerning a provider's rights and responsibilities as part of a network.

Provider-Sponsored Organization (PSO). A health care organization—established and organized, or operated, by a health care provider or a group of affiliated health care providers to arrange for the delivery, financing, and administration of health care—that meets requirements established by the Balanced Budget Act of 1997 and that has the authority to contract directly with Medicare.

purchasing alliances/coalitions/pools. Locally based, privately operated organizations that offer affordable group health coverage to businesses with fewer than 100 employees. Also known as purchasing pools, health insurance purchasing co-ops (HPCs), employer purchasing coalitions, or purchasing coalitions.

Q

QM committee. A managed care organization (MCO) committee responsible for oversight of the quality management program—including the setting of standards, review of data, feedback to providers, follow-up, and approval of sanctions—and for the quality of care delivered to members.

quality. In a managed care context, a managed care organization's (MCO's) success in providing health care and other services in such a way that plan members' needs and expectations are met.

quality management (QM). An organization-wide process of measuring and improving the quality of the health care provided by a managed care organization (MCO).

quality program. An organization-wide initiative to measure and improve the service and care provided by a managed care organization (MCO).

R

rate spread. The difference between the highest and lowest rates that a health plan charges small groups. The National Association of Insurance Commissioners (NAIC) Small Group Model Act limits a plan's allowable rate spread to 2 to 1.

rating. The process of calculating the appropriate premium to charge purchasers, given the degree of risk represented by the individual or group, the expected costs to deliver medical services, and the expected marketability and competitiveness of the managed care organization's (MCO's) plan.

reasonable and customary charges. Amounts charged by health care providers that are consistent with charges from similar providers for identical or similar services in a given locale.

rebate. A reduction in the price of a particular pharmaceutical obtained by a pharmacy benefit managements (PBM) plan from the pharmaceutical manufacturer.

recredentialing. Reexamination by a managed care organization (MCO) of the qualifications of a provider and verification that the provider still meets the standards for participation in the network.

relative value of services. See *relative value scale.*

relative value scale (RVS). A method used by managed care organizations (MCOs) of determining provider reimbursement that assigns a weighted value to each medical procedure or service. To determine the amount the MCO will pay to the physician, the weighted value is multiplied by a money multiplier. Also known as a relative value of services.

remittance advice. A report that outlines reimbursement data for multiple patient claims. The information provided varies by payer. Most reports will include basic information that outlines: patient account number; dates of service; the total/covered/allowed charges; the deductible and copay amounts due (from insured); contractual adjustments if applicable; and amount paid by the payer.

renewal underwriting. The process by which an underwriter reviews each year all the selection factors that were considered when the contract was issued, then compares the group's actual utilization rates to those the managed care organization (MCO) predicted to determine the group's renewal rate.

report card. A set of performance measures applied uniformly to different health plans or providers.

reserves. Estimates of money that an insurer needs to pay future business obligations.

Resource-Based Relative Value Scale (RBRVS). A method used by managed care organizations (MCOs) of determining provider reimbursement that attempts to take into account, when assigning a weighted value to medical procedures or services, all resources that physicians use in providing care to patients, including physical or procedural, educational, mental (cognitive), and financial resources.

retrospective authorization. Authorization to deliver health care service that is granted after service has been rendered.

revenues. The amounts earned from a company's sales of products and services to its customers.

risk-adjustment. The statistical adjustment of outcomes measures to account for risk factors that are independent of the quality of care provided and beyond the control of the plan or provider, such as the patient's gender and age, the seriousness of the patient's illness, and any other illnesses the patient might have. Also known as case-mix adjustment.

s

Secondary health insurance company. The secondary health insurance company is not the first payer of the patient's claims. The remaining claim balance will be sent to a secondary health insurance company, if provided, after payment is received by the primary health insurance company.

Section 1115 waivers. Waivers that states could obtain from the federal government that allowed them to set up managed care demonstration projects.

Section 1915(b) waivers. Waivers that states could obtain from the federal government that allowed them to restrict a Medicaid beneficiary's choice of providers by using a primary care case manager or other arrangement.

segments. See *market segments.*

self-funded plan. A health plan under which an employer or other group sponsor, rather than a managed care organization (MCO) or insurance company, is financially responsible for paying plan expenses, including claims made by group plan members. Also known as a self-insured plan.

self-insured plan. See *self-funded plan.*

senior market. A market segment that is comprised largely of persons over age 65 who are eligible for Medicare benefits.

service quality. A managed care organization's (MCO's) success in meeting the nonclinical customer service needs and expectations of plan members.

Sherman Antitrust Act. A federal act that established as national policy the concept of a competitive marketing system by prohibiting companies from attempting to (1) monopolize any part of trade or commerce or (2) engage in contracts, combinations, or conspiracies in restraint of trade. The Act applies to all companies engaged in interstate commerce and to all companies engaged in foreign commerce. See also *antitrust laws.*

Silent Preferred Provider Organization (PPO). A Silent PPO refers to a situation where, unbeknownst to its contracting physicians, a health plan "sells" or "rents" its PPO network of physicians to a third party (typically, a third-party administrator, insurance broker, smaller PPO, or self-insured employer) and that third party gets the advantage of whatever discount the health plan has negotiated with the physician.

small group. Although each managed care organization's (MCO's) size limit may vary, generally a group composed of 2 to 99 members for which health coverage is provided by the group sponsor.

specialty health maintenance organization (specialty HMO). An organization that uses a health maintenance organization (HMO) model to provide health care services in a subset or single specialty of medical care.

specialty HMO. See *specialty health maintenance organization.*

specialty services. Services that are provided by independent, specialty organizations rather than by the managed care organization (MCO) providing the basic health plan.

specific stop-loss coverage. See *individual stop-loss coverage.*

staff model HMO. A closed-panel health maintenance organization (HMO) whose physicians are employees of the HMO.

stale claim. A health care claim submitted by a physician practice after the health plan's allowable claims submission time limit.

standard community rating. A type of community rating in which an MCO considers only community-wide data and establishes the same financial performance goals for all risk classes. Also known as pure community rating.

standard of care. A diagnostic and treatment process that a clinician should follow for a certain type of patient, illness, or clinical circumstance.

Stark laws. See *Ethics in Patient Referrals Act.*

statutory solvency. An insurer's ability to maintain at least the minimum amount of capital and surplus specified by state insurance regulators.

stop-loss insurance. A type of insurance coverage that enables provider organizations or self-funded groups to place a dollar limit on their liability for paying claims and requires the insurer issuing the insurance to reimburse the insured organization for claims paid in excess of a specified yearly maximum.

structural integration. The unification of previously separate providers under common ownership or control.

structure measures. Health care quality indicators related to the nature and quality of the resources that a managed care organization has available for patient care.

subauthorization. The authorization of one health care service concurrently with the authorization of another service. For example, an authorization for hospitalization may cover surgery, anesthesia, pathology, and radiology performed during the hospitalization.

subsidiary. A company that is owned by another company, its parent.

super bill or patient charge slip. A form used by a physician practice to record services rendered by a physician or health care professional during the patient encounter. This form typically lists all the diagnostic, service, procedural, and other related codes that can be performed in the office.

surplus. The amount that remains when an insurer subtracts its liabilities and capital from its assets.

T

termination provision. A provider contract clause that describes how and under what circumstances the parties may end the contract.

termination with cause. A contract provision, included in all standard provider contracts, that allows either the managed care organization (MCO) or the provider to terminate the contract when the other party does not live up to its contractual obligations.

termination without cause. A contract provision that allows either the managed care organization (MCO) or the provider to terminate the contract without providing a reason or offering an appeals process.

third party administrator (TPA). A company that provides administrative services to managed care organizations (MCOs) or self-funded health plans.

treatment codes. See *diagnostic and treatment codes*.

TRICARE. A health care plan, available to more than 6 million military personnel and their families, which is administered by private contractors who are selected for participation through a competitive procurement process. TRICARE offers members three plan options: TRICARE Prime (a capitated health maintenance organization [HMO] with nominal premiums and copayments), TRICARE Extra (a preferred provider organization [PPO] with standard CHAMPUS deductibles), and TRICARE Standard (the current fee-for-service CHAMPUS plan with provider choice and no premiums). See also *Civilian Health and Medical Program of the Uniformed Services*.

U

underwriting. The process of identifying and classifying the risk represented by an individual or group.

underwriting impairments. Factors that tend to increase an individual's risk above that which is normal for his or her age.

underwriting manual. A document that provides background information about various underwriting impairments and suggests the appropriate action to take if such impairments exist.

underwriting requirements. Requirements, sometimes relating to group characteristics or financing measures, that managed care organizations (MCOs) at times impose in order to provide health care coverage to a given group and that are designed to balance a health plan's knowledge of a proposed group with the ability of the group to voluntarily select against the plan (antiselection).

usual, customary, and reasonable (UCR) fee. The amount commonly charged for a particular medical service by physicians within a particular geographic region. UCR fees are used by traditional health insurance companies as the basis for physician reimbursement.

utilization management (UM). Managing the use of medical services to ensure that a patient receives necessary, appropriate, high-quality care in a cost-effective manner.

utilization review (UR). The evaluation of the medical necessity, efficiency, and/or appropriateness of health care services and treatment plans.

utilization review committee. Committee that reviews utilization issues brought to it by the medical director, often approving or reviewing policy regarding coverage, reviewing utilization patterns of providers, and approving or reviewing the sanctioning process against providers.

utilization review organization (URO). External reviewers who assess the medical appropriateness of suggested courses of treatment for patients, thereby providing the patient and the purchaser increased assurance of the appropriateness, value, and quality of health care services.

V

value added network (VAN). A private network provider (sometimes called a turn-key communications line) that is hired by a health plan or physician practice to facilitate electronic data interchange (EDI) or provide other network services. Contemporary value added network providers now focus on offering EDI translation, encryption, secure e-mail, management reporting, and similar extra services for their customers.

variances. The differences obtained from subtracting actual results from expected or budgeted results.

W

withhold. A percentage of a provider's payment that is "held back" during the plan year to offset or pay for any cost overruns for referral or hospital services. Any part of the withhold not used for these purposes is distributed to providers.

workers' compensation. A state-mandated insurance program that provides benefits for health care costs and lost wages to qualified employees and their dependents if an employee suffers a work-related injury or disease.

workers' compensation indemnity benefits. Benefits that replace an employee's wages while the employee is unable to work because of a work-related injury or illness.

Page numbers in italic refer to figures or forms (f) and tables (t).

A

Accounts receivable aging reports, 3–4
Accounts receivables
    benchmarks for, 13
    likelihood of recovery of, *f14*
    remedies for problems with, 14
Adjustment rates, 4
Adjustments
    for collections, 4
    procedures for, 20–21
Administrative law judges (ALJs), 91
Advance Beneficiary Notice (ABN), 85, *f87*
Antikickback Statute, 45
Appeal letters, 80, *f81*
Appeals process, 80–83
    arbitration and, 82
    level 1 for, 81–82
    level 2 for, 82
    level 3 for, 82
    for Medicare, 90–92, *t90*
    software for, 79–80
    urgent review level for, 81
Arbitration, of appeals, 82–83
Assessment. *See* Self-assessment

B

Back office managed care matrix, *t98*
Balance billing, 53–57
Billing and collections operations
    assigning responsibilities, 31
    balance billing and, 53–57
    coding and, 38
    collection success analysis form for, *f52*
    establishing collection goals for, 51–53
    establishing fees for, 33–37
    establishing policies for, 33–37
    flowchart for, *f32*
    hiring staff for, 31–33
    identifying roles, 31
    training for, 37
    See also Payments

Billing clerks, patient encounters and, 10–11
Bonus plans, 38
Business office functions, *f35*

C

Capitation payment systems, 95, 100
   monitoring utilization of, 99
   verifying coverage for, 97
Carve-outs, fee-for-service, 99–100
Case rates, 99–100
Cash flows, tracking, 28
Cash handling, assessment of, 27–28
Cash payments, discounts for, 43–47
Central business office managers, as leaders, 15–16
Charge captures, assessment of, 23–26
Civil Monetary Penalties Law, 45
Claims
   clean (*see* clean claims)
   denied (*see* denied claims)
   electronic, 65, 76–77
   false, 93–94
   paper, 65
   payer follower-up for, 65
   processing, 65
   processing flowchart for, *f67*
   rejected, 77–79
   transmission of, 65
   unpaid, 77–79
"Claim-scrubber" software, 18, 64, 65
Clean claims
   for Medicare, 89–90
   obstacles to, *t69*
   processing flow chart for, *f67*
   submitting, 63–68
CMS-1500 claim form, 54, 89
Coding
   assessment of procedures for, 28–29
   basic knowledge about, 38
Collection letters, 70
Collection levels, assessment of, 14–15
Collection operations. *See* Billing and collections operations
Collection policies, 36–37
Collection referrals, 20
Collections, 66
Collections adjustments, 4
Collectors, performance standards for, 37
Compliance plans, assessment of, 26
Computer systems
   establishing electronic claims filing, 18
   reviewing, 17–18
   training for, 19
   upgrading, 18

Copayments
    collecting, 21–22, 47–49
    confirming, 47–49
    importance of, 49–50

D

Defined contribution plans. *See* Health Reimbursement Accounts (HRAs),
    collecting from
Denied claims, 66
    appealing, 79
    follow-up system for, 77–79
    software for, 79–80
Discounted fee-for-service, 99
Discounts, for cash payments, 43
    federal laws governing, 45

E

Education, patient, assessment of, 22
Electronic claims filing, establishing, 18
Electronic Data Interchange (EDI) transactions, Medicare, 92–93
Electronic submissions, 76–77
Encounter forms, 42
Encounters. *See* Patient encounters
Explanation of benefits (EOB), 75

F

Facilities, physical, assessment of, 29–30
False Claim Act, 45
False claims, 93–94
Fee-for-service payment systems, 95
Fees
    establishing, 33–37
    reductions of, 46
Fee schedules, Medicare, calculation of, 88–89
Finance charges, 56–57
Financial agreements, sample form for, *f44*
Flash reports, 23, *f24, f25*
Follow-ups, payer, 65
Fraud, 93–94
Front office functions, *f34*
Front office managed care matrix, *t96*
Front office staff, 8–11

G

Goals, establishing collection, 51–53
Grievances, filing, 83

H

Health Reimbursement Accounts (HRAs), collecting from, 51
Health Savings Accounts (HSAs), collecting from, 50–51
High-deductible plans, collecting from, 50

I

Incentives, 38
Income statements, 3
Incorrect payments, identifying, 75–76
Insurance, patient, verifying, 62–63
Insurance commissions, state, filing grievances with, 83
Insurance specialists
   patient encounters and, 11
   questions for collection levels for, 15
Insurers. *See* Payers, insurance
Interest income, tracking, 74
Internal controls, assessment of, 27–28
Internet, for patient insurance verification, 62–63

L

Leadership, 15–16
Lockbox services, 18–19, 28

M

Managed care contracts, assessment of, 29
Managed care matrix
   for back office, *t98*
   for front office, *t96*
Management reports
   assessment of, 23
   flash reports, *f24, f25*
Manuals, policies and procedures, 19–20
Medicare
   Advance Beneficiary Notice for, 85, *f87*
   appeals process for, 90–92, *t90*
   clean claims for, 89–90
   Electronic Data Interchange transactions for, 92–93
   fraud and, 93–94
   policy changes for, 88
   services covered by, 85, *t86*
Medicare Appeals Council (MAC), 91–92
Medicare Exclusion Statute, 45
Medicare fee schedules, calculation of, 88–89

N

No shows, charging for, 57–58

O

Office functions, *f34, f35*
Office managers, as leaders, 15–16
Operational organization, improving, 16–17

P

Parallel payment systems, defined, 95
Patient education, assessment of, 22
Patient encounters
  billing clerks and, 10–11
  front office staff and, 8–11
  insurance specialists and, 11
  practice managers and, 9
  questions for reviewing, 7–8
  receptionists and, 9–10
Patient insurance
  using Internet for verifying, 62–63
  verifying, 62
Payer follow-up, 65
Payer profiles
  developing, 68–73
  forms for, *f71, f72*
Payers, insurance
  charting performance of, 76
  dealing with slow, 73–75
Payments
  best time for collecting, 41–43
  establishing policies for, 33–37
  identifying incorrect, 75–76
  posting, 66
  See also billing and collections operations
Payment systems, 95
  front office matrix tool for, *t96*
  matrix tool for, 95
Performance standards, for collectors, 37
Personnel training, assessment of, 19
Physical facilities, assessment of, 29–30
Physicians, involvement of, in assessments, 3
Policies and procedures manuals, assessment of, 19–20
Practice managers, patient encounters and, 9
Prebilling protocols, 64
Price-fixing, 36
Professional courtesies, 20, 46
Prompt pay laws, 74

Q

Qualified independent contractors (QICs), 90–91

R

Rebilling fees, 57
Receptionists
  patient encounters and, 9–10
  payment policies and, 41–42
Refund requests, 20
Rejected claims, handling, 77–79

S

Self-assessment
  of accounts receivables, 13–14
  of adjustment process, 20–21
  of cash handling, 27–28
  of charge captures, 23–26
  checklist for, *t2*
  of coding procedures, 28–29
  of collection levels, 14–15
  of compliance plans, 26
  of computer systems, 17–19
  of copayment collections, 21–22
  of departmental direction and leadership, 15–16
  documents for, 3–4
  gathering data for, 1
  of internal controls, 27–28
  involving physicians in, 3
  of managed care contracts, 29
  of management reports, 23
  of operational organization, 16–17
  of patient education, 22
  of patient encounters, 7–11
  of personnel training, 19
  of physical facilities, 29–30
  of policies and procedures manuals, 19–20
  of staffing levels, 22
Self-pay, 43
  principles for collecting, 49
Slow insurance payers
  dealing with, 73–75
  ways to bills and collect from, 73
Staffing levels, assessment of, 22
Standards, performance, for collectors, 37
State insurance commissions, filing grievances with, 83
Statements
  pros and cons of sending, 56
  to third-party insurance companies, 66

T

Training, 19

U

Unpaid claims, handling, 77–79
Usury laws, 57

W

Waivers, 46
Write-offs, 20, 21

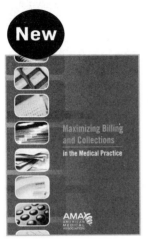
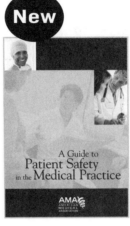
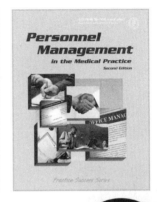
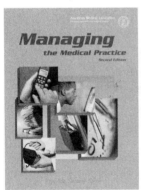
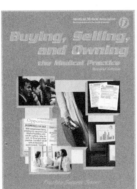
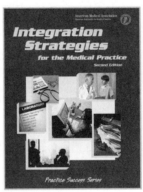
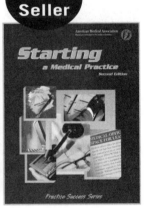
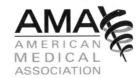